Halothane & Muscle Dysfunction

Navya

First Printing, 2024

CONTENTS.

Page.

INTRODUCTION.

Purpose of our Study.

The investigations to be presented in this book arose from studies on the respiration of mitochondria isolated from pig skeletal muscle. These animals developed the syndrome of Malignant Hyperthermia after exposure to halothane - a halogenated hydrocarbon us3d as an inhalation anaesthetic agent.

In our laboratory, Berman (1969) found that mitochondria, isolated from muscle of susceptible pigs, after exposure to halothane, exhibited markedly diminished oxygen uptake when NADH-linked substrates were oxidised. This was of particular interest, since in this syndrome there is a striking stimulation of muscle Glycogenolysis and accumulation of lactate (Berman et al 1970). This

— —

could be partly explained by the inhibition of NADH-linked mitochondrial respiration. However, succinate oxidation did not appear to be affected (Berman 1969). These findings were in agreement with those of Cohen et al (1969) and Miller et al (1970), who had observed the same inhibitory pattern of halothane whilst studying rat liver mitochondria.

Further studies in this laboratory have revealed a similar inhibitory action of halothane on mitochondria isolated from rat and normal porcine skeletal muscle at concentrations reached during general anaesthesia. In

preliminary .../

preliminary experiments, beef heart mitochondria have been observed to be similarly affected (Berman _et al_ 1970). This finding has been confirmed by Harris _et al_ (1971).

We hoped that a study on the effect of halothane on mitochondrial respiration would provide some insight into the mode of action of halogenated compounds. The fact that the inhibition was reversible and was localised in a specific section of the electron transport chain was of particular interest (Cohen 1969). We had a challenging project in trying to locate the site and mode of inhibition that was being exerted. Halothane might also serve as a probe of mitochondrial function, and the reversibility of its action could be related to conformational changes occurring within the membrane and protein structures.

The preparation of mitochondria from beef heart was chosen for a number of reasons. Beef heart mitochondria have been extensively employed in the study of intracellular respiration since the method was first developed by Keilin (1929). Subsequently, Keilin and Hartree (1949) 'standardised' the preparation, from which they could isolate a modified respiratory particle, capable of electron transport from NADH and succinate to molecular oxygen. This modified particle was nonphosphorylating, as it could not synthesise ATP. In addition, there are relatively few proteolytic enzymes in beef heart mitochondria, and the number of dehydrogenases is less than those present in mitochondria of other tissues, and thus the electron transfer system is assumed to be fairly stable in these mitochondria.

The alternative pathways for NADH oxidation that have been discovered in mitochondria of mammalian liver and bacteria are apparently absent from heart mitochondria. A relatively high yield of mitochondria was needed, and in this regard the most feasible methods were those for beef heart. Moreover, beef hearts were readily available.

The Mitochondrion.

(mitos: thread; chondros: grain.)

Structure.

Mitochondria were first identified at the turn of the present century. Supravital staining with Janus Green introduced by Michaelis, proved that the mitochondria of living cells could bring about oxidation and reduction changes in a dye. Mitochondria stained with this and other dyes can be detected with the light microscope, but rapid advance in their study came after the advent of the electron microscope. The particles may very in size, shape and number in different cells, but their ultra-structure is sufficiently characteristic for them to be identified as an individual class of cellular organelles in tissue of man, in protozoa and in fungi. They are localised in the cytoplasm and may vary in number from several hundred to a thousand per animal cell, depending on its location and function. They have an elongated, ellipsoid shape (Fig.1.) being 1,5μ by 0,5μ, with an average volume of $0,8\mu^3$.

It has been realised for many years that vitally important functions reside within the mitochondrion - in particular that of electron transport coupled to the trapping of energy liberated by the reactions of oxidative

phosphorylation .../

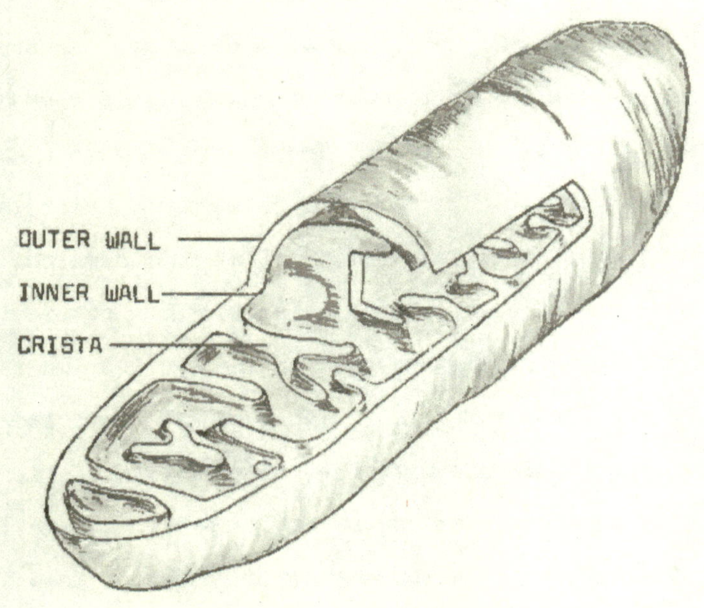

Fig. 1. SCHEMATIC REPRESENTATION OF THE MITOCHONDRION.

(Lehninger 1966)

phosphorylation - these functions continue to be the subject of intensive investigation and controversy. Albeit, they have proved excellent models for the study of phenomena of biological membranes. In the following discussion, those concepts and ideas relevant to the present investigation will be presented.

The mitochondrial organelle comprises two separable membrane systems, the outer boundary membrane and the inner boundary membrane. Together they form a barrier that can control the movement of ions and molecules into the mitochondrial interior. The inner membrane is convoluted to form tubular cristae. Each crista is closed on its interior end and open on the end that is continuous with the inner membrane. The lumen of the cristae are likewise continuous with the intermembrane space, although indications are that the outlet is extremely small and may limit the passage between the two spaces. Some cristae, e.g. those in canary heart muscle, are fused on their inner end, forming anastomoses, and are thus continuous to one another.

It is possible to distinguish the spaces within the mitochondrial membranes (Fig. 2.) : (a) lumina of the cristae, (b) intermembrane space, which lies between the inner and outer boundary membranes, and (c) matrix, the space between the cristae.

The .../

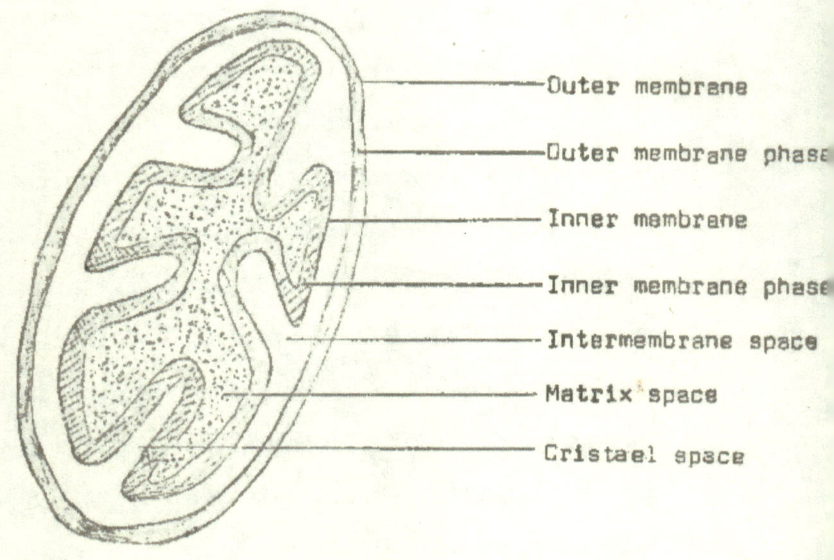

Fig. 2 The mitochondrion
(Klingenberg 1970)

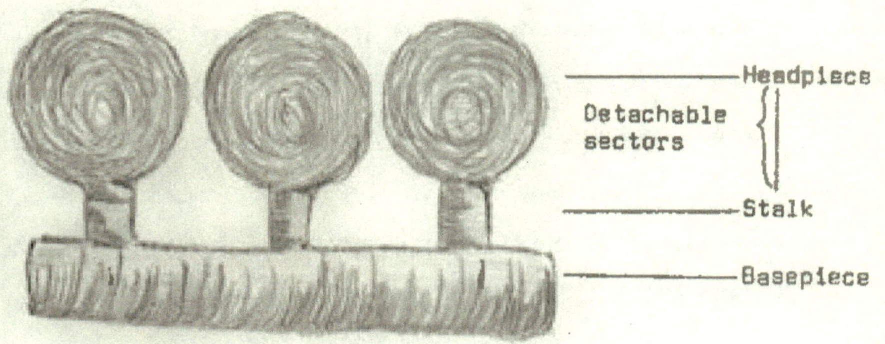

Fig. 3. Adjacent tripartite repeating units
(Green 1970)

The inner and outer membranes are separable by physical means and apparently have different properties, functions, and chemical composition. The outer membrane is more easily penetrated by small molecules, e.g. sucrose, and thus the intermembrane space is often referred to as the Sucrose Permeable Space (Klingenberg 1970). Components of the respiratory chain are absent from the outer membrane, the lipid content of which differs from that of the inner membrane. The inner membrane contains all the components of the respiratory chain, and is able to perform oxidative phosphorylation and is subject to respiratory control. Thus a membrane reflects the properties and functions of its components.

In 1956, Crane, Glenn and Green disrupted mitochondria to obtain two fragments, one of which appeared to be a portion of the external double membrane and of the cristae, whilst the second no longer possessed characteristics of the double membrane. The latter fragment, capable only of electron transport, was given the initials ETP, and the former, capable of electron transport and oxidative phosphorylation, was called ETP_H, H referring to the particle's capability of coupling phosphorylation to electron transport (Green 1962).

CAC Oxidation .../

	*CAC Oxidation	*ET	*OP
Mitochondria	+	+	+
ETP_H	-	+	+
ETP	-	+	-

*ET: Electron Transfer.

*OP: Oxidative Phosphorylation.

*CAC: Citric Acid Cycle.

The conversion of mitochondria to electron transport particles was quantitative, 80% of the dry weight of sonicated mitochondria accounted for ETP, implying that the mitochondria could be regarded as a polymer of repeating units.

Green et al (1970) have since characterised the inner membrane as consisting of macrotripartite repeating units (Fig. 3), readily visualised in negatively stained specimens (Fernandez-Moran et al 1964). These repeating units are believed to be the fundamental particle of controlled respiration and energy conservation. The units of the inner mitochondrial membrane have a molecular weight of 8-9 x 10^5 daltons, and are each composed of a basepiece, concerned with the 2-dimensional nesting of the repeating units, a stalk and a headpiece with sizes 5 x 10^5, 0,25 x 10^5, 3 x 10^5(daltons) respectively, (MacLennan

1968, Kopaczyk 1968). Protein accounts for 70% of the total mass, whilst the rest consists of lipid and phospholipid.

Two categories of protein have been isolated from the basepieces. The first are enzymes concerned with oxidative phosphorylation and other catalytic functions. The second group is non-catalytic and concerned with membrane biogenesis and ultrastructure; these proteins could exert a controlling influence on the catalytic group.

Analytical data indicate the basepiece to consist of not less than two molecules of non-catalytic protein (M.Wt. 60 000), five molecules of catalytic protein (M.Wt. 25 000), and three hundred molecules of phospholipid. Lipid is associated largely, if not exclusively, with the basepiece (Green 1963). Most of this lipid (95%) is phospholipid with minimal neutral lipid. Fatty acids present are generally highly unsaturated. The phospholipid is present as phosphatidyl choline, phosphatidyl ethanolamine, and cardiolipin. Pure phospholipid is thought to be capable of inducing _de novo_ membrane formation in an isolated system. The nature of the lipid of the membrane is relevant to properties, such a permeability.

There is a possibility that lipid forms a continuous

phase .../

phase extending from one repeating unit to the next, within the inner mitochondrial membrane continuum. It is feasible that the hydrophobic part of this lipid phase could contain the 'mobile' molecules, e.g. water insoluble CoQ and Cyt.c., the latter being known to bind electrostatically to phospholipid. Green's view, not accepted by all investigators, is that Cyt. c. could bind electrostatically to the charged phospholipid heads lining the surface of the cristael membrane, and thus move over the surface, fulfilling its function as an electron acceptor (Fig.4). In this way phospholipid could provide a bridge between the aqueous and non-aqueous phases. Albeit, the high percentage of phospholipid must have some bearing on membrane function.

The outer membrane of the mitochondrion, as has also the plasma membrane of erythrocytes, contains repeating units without projecting sectors, which correspond to the basepiece of the macrotripartite repeating units. These units in the outer membrane are designated monopartite.

Mitochondrial Function.

There are appropriate physical and chemical methods for separating the boundary and cristael membranes, and isolating the repeating units. Studies on such preparations are able to pinpoint in which membranes and in

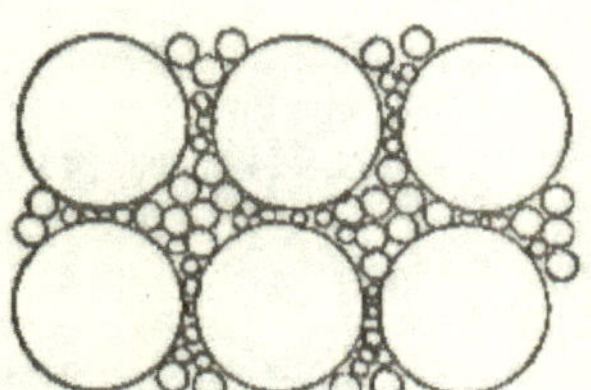

Fig. 4. Surface View of the Inner Boundary Membrane.

(Vanderkooi *et al* 1970).

which sector thereof the mitochondrial enzymes are located. Packed isolated mitochondria from heart and insect flight muscle have a membrane surface area of 50 square metres per ml; an impressive indication of the high proportion of membrane-bound reactions (Klingenberg 1970).

There is general agreement that the electron transfer chain and its enzymes, with the exception of certain dehydrogenases, are located in the basepieces of the inner membrane (Green _et al_ 1968, Allaman _et al_ 1968, and Schnaitman _et al_ 1968). It has also been demonstrated that succinate and NADH and their respective dehydrogenases interact with the respiratory chain at the inner or matrix face of the inner membrane (Harris 1967, Lee 1963). Cyt.c. on the other hand, seems to be located on the face of the inner membrane, bordering on the intermembrane space (Lee 1968, Palmieri 1967, Vanderkooi 1970). Chance _et al_ (1970) have observed that Cyt.c. present in intact mitochondria is reduced 100% by added $K_3Fe(CN)_6$, which is unable to penetrate the inner membrane. Cyt.c. must, therefore, be readily available on the membrane surface.

The isolated inner membrane-matrix complex of Schnaitman (1968), which consists of inner membrane and matrix only, can be prepared without solubilisation of NADH or NADPH dehydrogenases. This suggests that these enzymes are located within the mitochondrial matrix. However,

if .../

if the cristael orifice is as small as is believed, it is possible that the enzymes are trapped in the intermembrane space enclosed within folds of the cristae, and were not solubilised for this reason. Smoly (1970) was not able to exclude the possibility that the citric acid cycle enzymes and other enzymes are housed within this lumen. This hypothesis is supported by the electron micrographs of Korman _et al_ (1970), in which they have identified a paracrystalline structure, associated with the basepieces, which is possibly an array of such enzymes.

However, the controversy that existed as to the localisation of enzymes of the citric acid cycle and of fatty acid oxidation (Green 1966, Lardy 1969) seems to have been resolved (Van Dam 1971): these enzymes are located in the matrix of the mitochondria. There is, thus, a continual flux of metabolites between the exterior and the matrix space, from which the electron transfer chain draws its reducing source (Klingenberg 1970).

FIG. .../

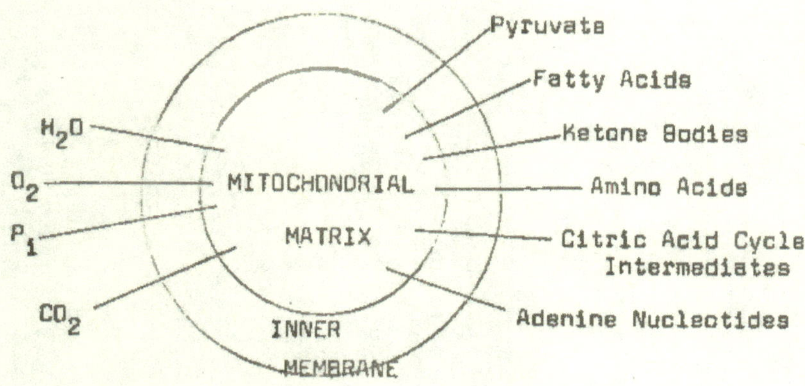

Fig. 5. The Metabolic Flux Through the Mitochondrial Membrane.(Klingenberg 1970).

Together with the evidence of Mitchell (1969), it is reasonable to assume that there is a loop-like arrangement of components of the electron transfer chain within the inner membrane structure, the pathway of reducing equivalents being from the matrix, or substrate donor side, to the intermembrane face and back (Smoly 1970). See Fig. 6.

Fig. 6..../

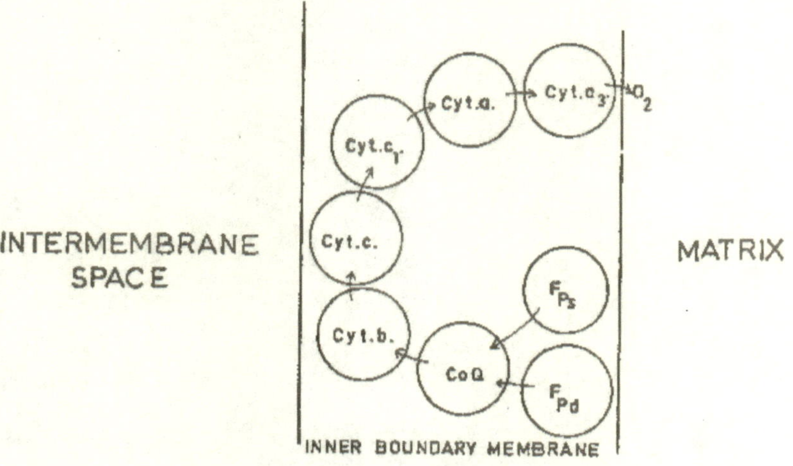

Fig. 6. Diagrammatic localisation of Components of the Electron Transport Chain Within the Inner Mitochondrial Membrane.

The stalk and headpiece portions of the tripartite units of the mitochondrion (Fig. 3) are thought to be active in ATP synthesis, since the headpiece has been found to consist mainly of ATPase (Kagawa et al 1966). The stalk also seems to be somehow related to the synthesis of ATP. However, in spite of developments which have enabled the various functions of the intact mitochondrion to be accurately mapped, it is still not possible to define whether the intermediate stages of energy conservation from electron transport are chemical

(Lipmann .../

(Lipmann 1946, Slater 1953), chemiosmotic (Mitchell 1961), or conformational (Boyer 1965, Harris *et al* 1968, Slater 1969).

The Respiratory Chain.

The early work of MacMunn, Keilin, Weiland and Warburg on the components of the respiratory chain has been reviewed by Lehninger (1965). The electron transfer chain (Figs. 7(a) & 7(b)) is composed of a system of sequential oxidations and reductions along an electropotential gradient. The chain itself is composed of two flavoprotein enzymes and four cytochromes, which together constitute the protein fraction. In addition, there is a non-protein component, ubiquinone and non-haem iron (NHI), which is that iron not bound to the porphyrin moeities of the cytochromes.

The two flavoprotein enzymes, NADH dehydrogenase (F_{Pd}) and succinic dehydrogenase (F_{Ps}), link the main substrate sources to the rest of the respiratory chain. Both enzymes contain flavin as a prosthetic group. F_{Pd} has flavin mononucleotide (FMN) and F_{Ps} has flavin adenine dinucleotide (FAD). Enzymatic and non-enzymatic reductions of the flavoproteins are characterised by the appearance of a transient electrun paramagnetic resonance signal, and absorption bands in the range 550 - 700 nm. This is consistent with the reduction occurring via two

consecutive .../

Fig. 7(a). Schematic Representation of Mitochondrial Electron Transport and Oxidative Phosphorylation.

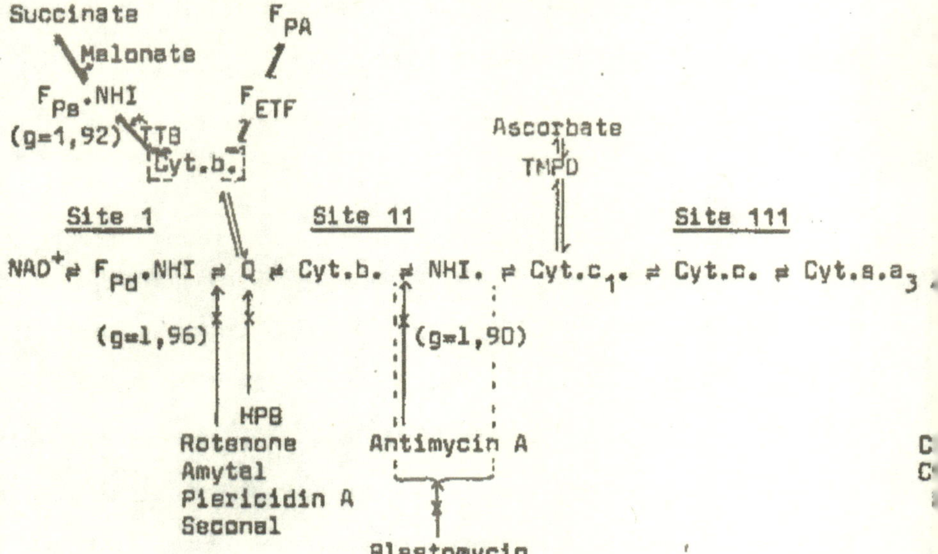

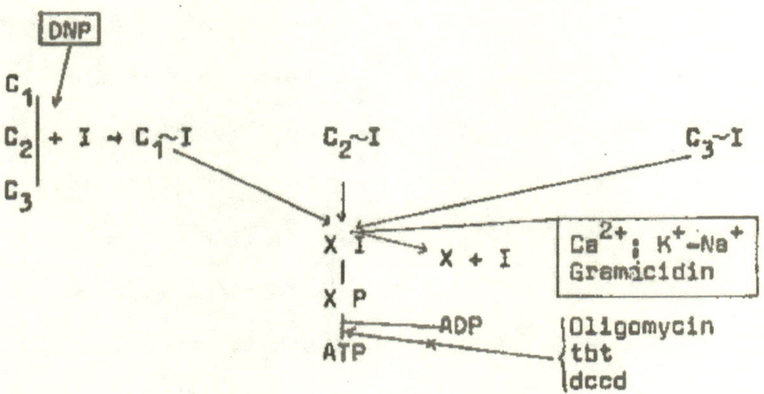

F_{Pd} :NADH Dehydrogenase

F_{Ps} :Succinate Dehydrogenase

F_{PA} : Fatty Acyl CoA Dehydrogenase

F_{ETF} :Electron Transfer Flavoprot

tbt :tributyltin

dccd :dichlorocyclohexylcarbodi-i

DNP :1,4 Dinitrophenol

TTB :4,4,4,-trifluoro-1-(2-thienyl)-1,3-butadione

HPB :2,3-dimethoxy-5-hydroxy-6-phytyl-1,4,-benzoquinone

☐ :Uncoupler

Fig. 7(b). The Respiratory Chain as it is Believed to Occur in Mammalian Mitochondria.

(Van Dam *et al*. 1971.)

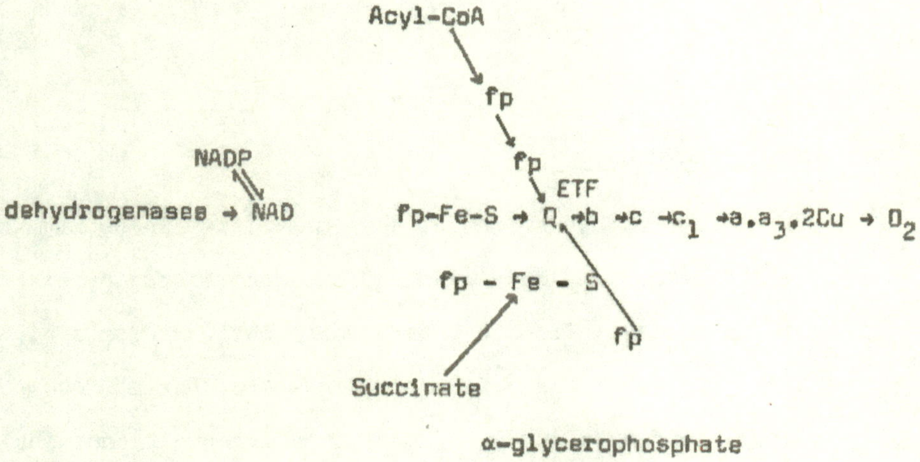

Acyl-CoA

fp

fp

NADP

ETF

dehydrogenases → NAD fp-Fe-S → Q → b → c → c_1 → a.a_3.2Cu → O_2

fp - Fe - S

fp

Succinate

α-glycerophosphate

consecutive one-electron transfers. In the course of the reaction the isoalloxazine ring system becomes reduced:-

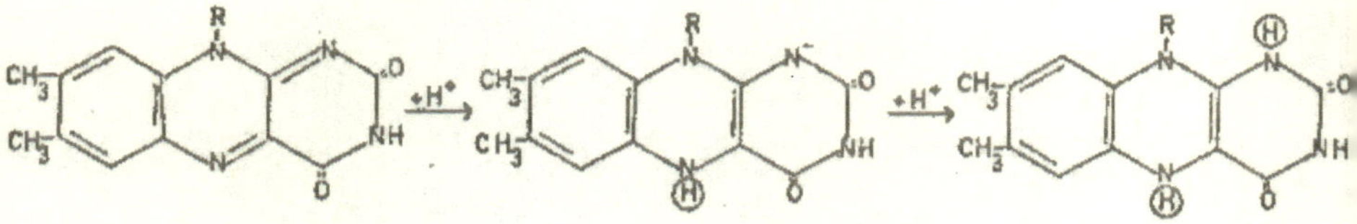

The Cytochromes.

These may be defined as "enzymes" that employ haem as their co-enzyme. Both haem and chlorophyll occupy a vital role in electron transfer, each being derived from a porphyrin nucleus. Haem is a metal chelate, formed from protoporphyrin IX and iron, whereas chlorophyll contains magnesium in chlorin, a modified porphyrin ring.

The term cytochrome is applied to all those haemoproteins which act as electron carriers by engaging in a ferrous-ferric cycle. The different types of cytochromes have been empirically separated into four classes: A, B, C, and D, on the basis of spectral appearance of their pyridine haemochromogen derivatives. (See Appendix.)

In addition to these proteins, there are two other protein-bound redox entities. Non-haem iron (NHI) is linked to the NADH and succinate dehydrogenases, and lies

between .../

between cytochrome b and c. Copper is associated with cytochrome a. and can exist in the cupric or cuprous form.

Ubiquinone.

This compound is also often referred to as Benzoquinone or Coenzyme Q (CoQ). It is capable of interacting with flavoproteins and with cytochrome b. and is thought, therefore, to be the convergence point of hydrogen equivalents from succinate and NADH, Acetyl CoA and α glycerophosphate, (Fig. 7(b)). However, its exact siting is controversial, and there are indications that it may exist on a side chain. This suggestion will be considered further in discussion later.

The plastoquinones have an analogous carrier role in photosynthetic transport, and differ from ubiquinones in that they have shorter side chains.

NADH-Cytochrome Reductase.

As the studies to be reported here show that halothane and other halogenated hydrocarbons have a specific inhibitory action on this portion of the mitochondrial respiratory system, it will be considered in some detail. It remains the most controversial and least understood complex within the electron transport chain.

A portion of the electron transport chain, linking NADH and the cytochromes, was first separated as two

Complexes .../

Complexes (I & III) by Hatefi _et al_ (1961, 1962). Complex I, or NADH-CoQ Reductase, catalyses the reaction:

$$NADH + CoQ + H^{+} \longrightarrow NAD^{+} + CoQH_2$$

Complex III or $CoQH_2$ - Cyt.c. links CoQ with Cytochrome c., thus:

$$CoQH_2 + 2Cyt.c. (Fe^{3+}) \longrightarrow CoQ + 2Cyt.c. (Fe^{2+})$$

However, the system is not as simple as this, because of the presence of intermediate acceptors of the electrons as well as catalytic and structural protein moeities. The many methods described for isolating these discrete components in the unaltered state reflect the complexity of the technical problems, which is manifest too, in the consequent differences in reactivity with artificial and natural electron acceptors. These preparations are briefly outlined in Table 1 modified from Redfearn _et al_ (1964).

The fact that Sanadi's preparation (1965) reduces menadione, ferricyanide and Cyt.c. as well as CoQ, its natural acceptor, has led to disagreement as to whether his assumption that this is the natural enzyme, is, indeed, valid. In isolated mitochondria and submitochondrial fragments, structural restraints on the intact mitochondria may be disrupted, thus giving rise to such artificial systems. On the other hand, although outlined in various schemes, the cytochromes and CoQ have not been located

exactly .../

TABLE 1.

PREPARATIONS OF NADH DEHYDROGENASE COMPLEX.

	Enzyme	Investigator	Starting Material	Solubilisation Conditions	Preparation	Non-protein Moiety mμmoles	Approx. M.Wt.	Substrate	Acceptor	Inhibitors.
1.	*NADH Cyt.c. Reductase	Hatefi et al (1961)	Beef heart mitochondria according to P.Blair (1967)		Red green separation of Cytochromes, Dialysis DOC, NH_3 Acetate fractionation.	0,97 total flavin 1,13 Cyt.b. 0,81 Cyt.c. + c_1 3,7 CoQ 14-16 NHI 0,3 - 0,35 mg. Lipid.		NADH	Cyt.c.	Antimycin A Rotenone 0,4mM Amytal (50%)
2.	NADH Cyt.c. Reductase	Mahler et al (1952)	Heart particles	Acid-ethanol $42^o - 44^oC$.		1 Flavin 4 Haem	80 000	NADH	Cyt.c.	
3.	NADH Cyt.c. Reductase	De Bernard (1957)	ETP	Acid-ethanol 43^oC.		1 Flavin 2 Haem		NADH	Cyt.c.	
4.	NADH Dehydrogenase	King et al (1962)	ETP - Keilin Hartree preparation.	Naja naja Venom 37^oC.		1 FMN 4 Fe	120 000	NADH	Cyt.c. DCIP $K_3Fe(CN)_6$	Unaffected by Antimycin A. (2μg/mg.protein) Amytal 5mM.
5.	NADH Dehydrogenase	Mackler, Huennekens et al (1963)	'DPNH oxidase'	Modification of De Bernard, Ethanol pH 4.8 43^oC Amm. sulfate fractionation		11 FMN 20 μatoms Haem		NADH	$K_3Fe(CN)_6$ DCIP, Cyt.c. FAD, FMN to a lesser extent.	pCMB 0,4mM Amytal (1mM) - little effect if any. Antimycin A 1 μg/ml.
6.	**NADH Dehydrogenase	Singer, Ringler et al (1963)	ETP ETP_H	Naja naja Venom 30^oC		1,23 FMN	550 000	NADH	$K_3Fe(CN)_6$	Amytal 3mM., Antimycin A. 10^{-6}M - both no effect.
7.	NADH Dehydrogenase	Chapman and Jagannathan (1963) King (1967)	ETP - Keilin Hartree preparation	Thiourea 0^oC Gives 2 fractions.		(1) 1,98 FMN 27,7 NHI (11) 4,83 FMN 49,1 NHI	200 000	NADH	$K_3Fe(CN)_6$ CoQ_2, 3,6,10' Cyt.c. Menadione, Vit. K_1	Amytal - no inhibition.

TABLE 1. (CONTINUED)

PREPARATIONS OF NADH DEHYDROGENASE COMPLEX.

	Enzyme	Investigator	Starting Material	Solubilisation Conditions.	Pre-paration	Non-protein Moeity mμmoles	Approx. M.Wt.	Sub-strate	Acceptor	Inhibitors.
8.	NADH Ubiquinone Reductase	Sanadi, Pharo *et al* (1968)	SP_{HL}	pH5,3 in ethanol, 43°C Gives 2 equal fractions.		1 FMN 4 NHI 5 Labile sulfate	90 000	NADH	$K_3Fe(CN)_6$, $CoQ_{1,6,10}$ Cyt.c. Menadione	CoQ_6 complete inhibition by Amytal and Rotenone, insensitive to Piericidin A. Menadione partially inhibited.

* Using NADH - Cyt.c. Reductase as starting material one can prepare:
(i) NADH - CoQ reductase which is equivalent to the enzyme of the intact particles described by Singer (1963). It is Amytal and Rotenone sensitive. (Hatefi (1962))
(ii) Reduced Coenzyme Q - Cyt.c. reductase (Rasieka et al (1964)). Sensitive to Antimycin A.

** The extract NADH - CoQ reductase (pH5,4, 95% ethanol at 43°C for 15 minutes) loses its characteristic properties of catalytic activities of the dehydrogenase and becomes highly catalytic towards CoQ_6, CoQ_{10}, and Cyt.c. It is inhibited by Amytal and Rotenone.

2 - 8 Soluble enzyme preparations.

exactly in the intact system. It is, therefore, feasible that these might 'move' about within the electron transfer chain. The reduction of Cyt.c. in Sanadi's preparation (1965) need not, therefore, be a result of the structural disarray of the system, but could be a natural reaction.

The localisation of Cytochrome c. has also been questioned by Nicholls (1964), who has shown a 2:1 stoichiometry between Cyt.a. and Cyt.c. respectively, suggesting that Cyt.a. redox reactions involve transfer of a single electron rather than an electron pair. The transfer of electron pairs to Cyt.a. has been used as an argument for its localisation within the electron transfer chain.

The high molecular weight form of the NADH Dehydrogenase ($NADH_2$: (acceptor) oxido reductase E.C. : 1.6.99.3) extracted by means of Phospholipase A (Salach et al 1967) is thought to possess properties similar to the enzyme present in the intact particles. However, it does not possess Ubiquinone Reductase activity unless subjected to acid-ethanol treatment. The lack of CoQ reductase activity in the purified dehydrogenase is likely to be related to the absence of lipids. Singer (1968) has shown that a brief digestion of the particles by cobra venom phospholipase leads to inactivation of the Rotenone-sensitive NADH-CoQ reaction. This inactivation

may .../

may be reversed by the addition of phospholipids. Prolonged incubation with phospholipase leads to irreversible inactivation. Other lipids, including CoQ_{10}, which may not be readily replaced, are lost.

The complete transformation of NADH dehydrogenase, an enzyme virtually devoid of CoQ reductase activity, into one which reduces long or short chain CoQ homologues, an activity in which it is inhibited by Amytal and Rotenone in the same manner as the soluble NADH-CoQ reductase of Phero and Sanadi (1968), strongly suggests that these CoQ reductase activities are not physiological, but emerge as a consequence of conformational changes in the protein. Other preparations do function as CoQ reductase with lipid present, and these could contain the physiologically intact enzyme.

Burstein et al (1971) have shown that the exposure of beef heart mitochondria to purified preparations of phospholipase A or phospholipase C results in losses of phosphorylation capacity, but respiration is not impaired. The system is protected by bovine serum albumin at low concentrations of either lipase. Exposure of submitochondrial particles to the phospholipases A and C impaired the rate of oxidation as well as phosphorylation. In addition, both lipases were more inhibitory to phosphorylation and to NADH oxidation than to succinate oxidation. Analysis of the NADH dehydrogenase activity after digestion with phospholipase C. revealed that it was still associated with the particles, but that NADH oxidase activity was lost. This phenomenon, which has previously been observed after digestion of particles with phospholipase A, (Machinist _et al_ 1965), points to a specific role of phospholipids in the NADH-CoQ_{10} segment of the respiratory chain.

Although the molar concentration of NADH dehydrogenase in mammalian mitochondria is at least an order of magnitude lower than that of any of the cytochromes (Klingenberg 1968), the high turnover number of the dehydrogenase means that it is not likely to become rate-limiting during the events of electron transport (Singer, 1968).

The NADH dehydrogenase extracted with phospholipase A at 30°C. and 37°C. is often designated form I, (Ringler _et al_ 1963), while form II is assigned to the preparations extracted by heating at 42 - 43°C., by acid-ethanol, or urea.

Form II is regarded by some workers as a relatively unmodified enzyme, preexisting as such in the mitochondrion, the differences in properties between the bound and extracted form being ascribed to the influence of the environment in the particle-bound state (Mackler _et al_, 1966, Pharo 1968, King 1966). Hatefi (1968) envisages the particulate enzyme as a complex of enzymes consisting

of .../

of flavoprotein, NHI protein and structural protein, dissociable by urea. The flavoprotein portion corresponds to form II. Tyler _et al_ (1965) gave experimental evidence for the existence of a separate flavoprotein and NHI protein. Gutman _et al_ (1970) has proposed a third interpretation, namely that the NADH dehydrogenase is a single enzyme composed of many polypeptide chains, the strained conformation being upheld by membrane structure. This would account for the numerous polypeptide forms which can be isolated after various treatments. Form II is thus one of many alternative products. One would expect, however, that other forms would also have been isolated.

Nevertheless, NADH dehydrogenase is a complex and unusual protein, and because of the controversy existing in this section of the electron transfer chain, arguments based on the possible sites of action of inhibitors cannot be rigorous. In approaching our system we accepted that CoQ may, or may not, be on the direct pathway from NADH to molecular oxygen. Also, it may, or may not, be directly coupled to NADH oxidation by NADH dehydrogenase. Similarly, there is the possibility that Cyt.c. may be directly coupled to the dehydrogenase (Storey 1967, Jeng _et al_ 1968).

Inhibitors of the NADH-CoQ segment of the Respiratory Chain.

There are three classes of inhibitors known to act

on .../

on this section of the chain, barbiturates (e.g. Amytal and Seconal); Rotenone, and Piericidin A (Hall et al 1966, Teeter et al 1969).

These inhibitors compete for the same site in the chain (Horgan et al 1968). With the aid of bovine serum albumin (BSA) and ^{14}C-labelled inhibitors it is possible to distinguish between two types of binding sites:

(a) Specific binding sites, defined as sites from which labelled Rotenone or Piericidin A are not removed by BSA. These sites are those responsive to inhibition in the NADH dehydrogenase-ubiquinone region.

(b) Unspecific binding sites in mitochondria and sub-mitochondrial particles from which these inhibitors are readily dissociated by BSA.

The specific binding site titre for Rotenone and Piericidin A is 1,5 - 2,0 moles/mole of NADH dehydrogenase in electron transport particles (ETP), but approached 1,0 in simpler particles, e.g. Complex I or I + III (Horgan et al 1968). Using Scatchard plots, a more precise value of 2,0 for ETP and 1,2 for Complex I was obtained (Gutman et al 1970). The tenacious binding at the specific sites is noncovalent and probably involves both lipid and protein. The fact that BSA is capable of partially reversing the inhibition at low concentrations of Piericidin A indicates that some non-specific binding

contributes .../

contributes to the observed inhibition.

The correlation between the content of NADH dehydrogenase and specific binding site titre suggests a role of the enzyme in Rotenone and Piericidin A binding. This is not supported by the fact that incubation with Phospholipase A solubilised all the dehydrogenase from ^{14}C-Rotenone-inhibited ETP without extracting any label. However, this treatment, as well as that by other protein-modifying reagents, causes extensive translocation of the labelled inhibitor to unspecific sites, whence it is removed by BSA (Horgan 1968). In further experiments, Gutman _et al_ (1970) have shown that prior binding of Piericidin A at the specific sites strongly inhibits solubilisation of the dehydrogenase and prevents the removal of specific binding sites by digestion with Phospholipase A. Apparently, Piericidin A is bound specifically at a locus close to the phospholipids, hydrolysed by phospholipase A, which may be involved in binding of the NADH dehydrogenase.

The dehydrogenase has also been modified with mersalyl. Purified preparations of membrane-free enzyme are altered by mersalyl as regards their substrate specificity and susceptibility to various inhibitors (Table 1). Mersalyl was chosen to modify the enzyme because it inhibits NADH oxidation in ETP, and has a

similar .../

similar effect on highly purified soluble preparations of the dehydrogenase (Tyler 1965). Treatment of ETP with 30µM mersalyl changed the binding of ^{14}C-Piericidin A and decreased the specific site titre to 1,2 (from 2,0). However, once Piericidin A is attached at its specific site, added mersalyl does not release it, although a modification of NADH dehydrogenase by this mercurial compound is still evident. These experiments support the hypothesis that the conformation of the NADH dehydrogenase as it exists within the mitochondrion in vivo is essential for optimal binding of Piericidin A, and that the flavoprotein may be one of the anchoring sites of Rotenone, Piericidin A and the barbiturates.

Although the effects of Rotenone, Piericidin A and Amytal are exerted in the same area, they differ in that the former inhibits electron transfer equally in the forward and ATP-supported reverse directions (Burgos et al 1965). Amytal, however, inhibits ATP-Pi exchange, whereas Piericidin A does not.

The purified ubiquinone reductase of Pharo and Sanadi et al (1968) is inhibited by Amytal and Rotenone. The latter exhibits an atypical biphasic curve with maximum inhibition when the ratio of Rotenone to enzyme-flavin is 1,0. Piericidin A and dicoumarol do not depress the activity of the purified reductase.

Piericidin A .../

Piericidin A is a highly specific inhibitor of NADH oxidase, which is inhibited 50% by 18pmoles/mg. protein and 100% by 36 pmoles/mg. Comparable inhibition of succinoxidase can only be achieved with 20 000 times this concentration of inhibitor. Vallin & Löw (1968) proposed that the effectiveness of the antibiotic is dependent on the redox state of CoQ, since the energy-dependent reduction of NAD^+ by succinate or TMPD was 10 times more sensitive to Piericidin A than was NADH oxidation.

Metabolic Effects of Halothane.

In 1956 halothane was introduced as a general anaesthetic agent, and has since become the most widely used inhalation anaesthetic compound. Approximately ten million doses are given annually in the world. Halogenated hydrocarbons employed for anaesthesia differ from ethers employed for a similar purpose, in their having an increased stability, pleasant smell, a non-irritant vapour, and higher boiling points (Halothane 50,2°C). The lack of volatility is compensated for by greater potency.

Halothane decomposes slowly on exposure to light with the formation of volatile acids. It is stable if stored in amber-coloured bottles, and thymol is usually added to retard decomposition.

The halogenated hydrocarbons containing bromine undergo changes in the body, as has been proved by the isolation of inorganic bromides in the urine and perspiration after administration of brominated hydrocarbons.

The degradation of halogenated hydrocarbons in general has been studied in some detail. Although most of the elimination of volatile halogenated hydrocarbons is via the lungs, it has been shown that *in vivo* hydrolysis

does .../

does take place. The saturated derivatives are less stable *in vivo* than the unsaturated ones, and two carbon compounds are more stable than single carbon compounds.

It has been demonstrated in man and animals that halothane labelled with Cl or C undergoes biotransformation. In dogs the molecule is disrupted at the C - Cl bond (Adriani 1968). The degradative reaction is accelerated by NADPH, and presumably occurs in the microsomes of the liver, and to a lesser extent, of the brain (Adriani 1968). Other evidence indicates that Br is removed in a similar manner. The resulting metabolites of halothane are a chloride, a bromide, and trifluoroacetic acid (Stier 1964). Determinations of trifluoroacetic acid in the urine indicate 10 - 20% breakdown of halothane in man.

Metabolic studies in man and animals prove that halothane has minimal effects on general metabolism. Some diminution (20%) in oxygen consumption during anaesthesia has been noted, but this has been attributed to diminished diaphragmatic and cardiac work when assisted ventilatory systems are employed. There is no evidence that depressed cellular respiration plays any part in producing anaesthesia. This point is of particular importance since, as will be shown, significant depression of mitochondrial respiration can be elicited at concentrations of halothane readily reached during

clinical .../

clinical anaesthesia.

The question which immediately arises is why such inhibition is not evident in the whole animal. This will be considered later in the discussion.

Objectives of the Investigation and Salient Findings Which Were Made.

In this study we investigated the inhibition, by halothane and other halogenated hydrocarbons, of the electron transport of mitochondria of beef heart and submitochondrial particles, to discover, if possible, whether this metabolic derangement was, in any way, related to the syndrome of Malignant Hyperthermia. We wished to establish, too, whether the inhibitory pattern in beef heart mitochondria was similar to that observed in other tissues. It was also our aim to determine the specificity of the inhibition for various sites within the mitochondrion, and to assess the importance of the structure of the membranes of this and other organelles in relation to the mode of inhibition. We also wanted to study the mechanism by which halogenated compounds in general were inhibitive, and thus determine if there was any relationship between the degree of halogenation and extent of inhibition. There is the possibility that the inhibition caused by these compounds depends on their lipid solubility.

The inhibition of beef heart mitochondria and submitochondrial particles by halothane was found to be similar to that observed by other workers in other tissues. The inhibition proved to be specific for NADH dehydrogenase and uncompetitive in type. The solubilised

enzyme .../

enzyme was not inhibited, from which it is evident that a requirement for effective inhibition by the halogenated hydrocarbons is that the enzyme be membrane-bound as it is normally present within the mitochondrion. The extent of inhibition of the particulate enzyme was related to the degree of halogenation of the inhibitory compound.

MATERIALS AND METHODS.

Mitochondria and submitochondrial particles (ETP) were prepared from beef heart. The respiration of these was studied, using various substrates, and followed either by measuring oxygen consumption polarographically, or by following the reduction of artificial electron acceptors spectrophotometrically.

Similar investigations were also made on NADH dehydrogenase preparations after solubilisation from their usual membrane-bound state.

Parallel experiments were made on these systems after addition of halothane or one of a series of chlorinated hydrocarbons.

Materials.

Antimycin A, α-ketoglutarate, ADP, malate, malonate, Rotenone, NADH, CoQ_6, CoQ_{10}, Menadione were obtained from Sigma Chemical Co.

Pyruvate, ADP, Cyt.c. (Horse heart, Grade I), β-NADH were purchased from Miles Seravac, Cape Town.

BSA was obtained from Pentex Incorporated, Illinois, U.S.A.

Amytal was from Lilly Laboratories, and halothane was obtained from Imperial Chemical Industries Ltd., London, and contained 0,1% thymol as preservative. In subsequent experiments no difference was discernible between the metabolic activity of freshly distilled halothane and the thymol-preserved compound. In all the experiments reported in this book, halothane preserved with thymol was employed.

All other chemical reagents used were of the highest analytical grade available.

Methods.

Preparation of Heavy Beef Heart Mitochondria. (Method 1.)
(A.Smith (1967), modified from Crane *et al* (1956) and Hatefi *et al* (1961)).

Beef heart was obtained within half an hour of slaughter, placed on ice, and all subsequent work conducted at 0° - $4^{o}C$.

Fat, blood clots, and connective tissue were removed, and the heart cut into ± 5 cm. cubes, and 300 gm batches passed through a meat grinder, with a plate with 4 mm holes.

The resultant mince, from 300 gms heart muscle, was added to 400 ml 0,25M sucrose, 0,01M tris-HCl pH 7,8. The pH was adjusted immediately to 7,5 ± 0,1 with 6M KOH or 2M tris. The neutralised minced heart was then poured on to a double layer of fine cheesecloth and squeezed free of the sucrose solution.

Two hundred gms of the resulting washed mince was suspended in 400 ml of 'sucrose solution' (0,25M sucrose, 0,01M tris, pH 7,8, containing 1mM tris-succinate and 0,2mM EDTA).

Subsequent processing was by one or other of the following procedures:

Either: (i) 50 ml aliquots of the above suspension were transferred to a glass homogenising vessel into which was inserted a loose fitting pestle, driven at

No. 7 speed on the scale of the Gallenkamp stirrer motor, with 2 passes of ± 15 seconds and two of 5 - 10 seconds. The final homogenate was readjusted to pH 7,8 by addition of 1M KOH or 2M tris.

Or: (ii) Two hundred gms of ground mince heart in 400 ml of sucrose solution were transferred to a 1 Litre Waring blendor, and either 1 ml 6M KOH or 3 ml 2M tris added. The blendor was run at maximum speed for 15 seconds, 1 ml 6M KOH then added, and the homogenisation continued for 5 seconds. The pH was finally adjusted to 7,8 with 1M KOH.

Unruptured muscle and nuclei were now removed from either homogenate by centrifuging at 1 200 x g (2 750 r.p.m.) for 20 minutes in a fixed angle rotor (No. 5,75) of the Sorvall Superspeed RC-2B centrifuge.

The supernatant was decanted and filtered through two layers of cheesecloth to remove granules of lipid. The pH was readjusted to 7,8 with 1M KOH and the suspension transferred to cellulose nitrate tubes, and spun in the No. 30 rotor of Beckman Spinco Model L centrifuge for 15 minutes at 26 000 x g (15 000 r.p.m.).

The resultant pellet consisted of (from above downwards):

(1) .../

(1) a light pinkish layer (LBHM),

(2) a buff to dark brown area (HBHM), the layer required, and

(3) a brown-black smudge not visible in all tubes.

The LBHM layer was removed by decanting 25 ml of the supernatant sucrose solution, agitating the remaining supernatant gently, to dislodge the LBHM, and the suspension then removed with a Pasteur pipette and discarded.

The second layer (HBHM) was dislodged with a glass rod, and 5 - 10 ml of sucrose solution added. The tube was gently shaken and the suspension removed with a Pasteur pipette. The pooled fractions were homogenised, using a tight fitting smooth teflon pestle in a glass vessel, and the Gallenkamp stirring apparatus (speed No. 7) with two passes of ± 5 seconds. The volume was brought to 100 ml and adjusted pH to 7,8. The HBHM suspension was spun as before for 25 minutes. The resultant pellet of homogeneous HBHM was homogenised, adjusted to pH 7,8, and centrifuged a third time for 15 minutes.

After the final spin, the pellet surface was washed with sucrose solution, the pellet dislodged, homogenised, and the pH adjusted as before. The protein concentration

was .../

was adjusted to 30 mg/ml. The resulting suspension of HBHM was kept on ice until used. Repeatable results were possible in this manner for up to one week.

Yield: 1 - 2 mgs protein/gm of starting material.

Although this preparation has been used by many workers for similar kinds of inhibitory studies on NADH dehydrogenase, anomalous results were obtained in preliminary studies of inhibition, being variable and unpredictable. The source of error was eventually traced to the presence of 1mM succinate in the "sucrose solution", variable quantities of which could be transferred into the reaction mixture, and, depending on the volume of HBHM suspension used, contribute to total oxygen consumption.

For this reason the preparation of Pharo et al (1966) which does not require succinate addition, was also tried. It had the further advantage of higher mitochondrial yield.

Preparation .../

Preparation of Heavy Beef Heart Mitochondria. (Method 2.)
(Pharo et al 1966)

Minced bovine heart muscle (prepared as before) was suspended in 200 gm portions in 500 ml of medium containing 0,25M sucrose, 13mM tris, 13mM K_2HPO_4 and 0,1mM EDTA, pH 7,8. This mixture was homogenised at 15-second intervals for 45 seconds at maximum speed in a 1 Litre Waring blendor.

The homogenate was centrifuged at 1 000 x g (2 500 r.p.m.) for 15 minutes in a Sorvall Superspeed RC-28 centrifuge. The supernatant was filtered through several layers of cheesecloth into a chilled beaker. The centrifugal deposit of muscle cells and nuclei was rehomogenised in 250ml of 0,25M sucrose containing 15mM K_2HPO_4 for 30 seconds. Such homogenisation is known to double the yield of mitochondria. The homogenate was centrifuged as before for 10 minutes. The combined supernatants were spun at 15 000 x g (13 100 r.p.m.) for 10 minutes in a No. 21 rotor of the Beckman Spinco Model L preparative ultracentrifuge. The pellet was suspended in a 0,25 sucrose and homogenised with a loose fitting teflon pestle. The pH was then adjusted to 7,8 with 1M tris. The suspension was spun at 26 000 x g (15 000 r.p.m.) for 60 minutes in the No. 30 rotor of the

Beckman .../

Beckman Centrifuge.

The mitochondrial pellet was suspended in 0,25 M sucrose at a protein concentration of 25 mg/ml and, if it was to be used for the preparation of submitochondrial particles, stored at - 20^{0}C. Otherwise it was stored on ice for use within one week.

Yield: 5 mg mitochondrial protein/gm of starting material.

Preparation of Submitochondrial Particles. (ETP).

(Sanadi et al 1967)

The mitochondrial suspension was frozen in solid CO_2, then thawed and the pH adjusted to 7,4. The mitochondria were now disrupted by exposure to sonic oscillation with an MSE-type sonifier operating at maximum power output for 5 minutes. The head of the sonifier was lowered into the vessel so that the arm was a few mm below the surface of the preparation. The vessel containing the mitochondrial suspension was immersed in a bath of 50% ethylene glycol at - 10^{0}C. In this way the temperature of the sonified particles did not rise above 2^{0}C.

Unbroken mitochondria and large particles were removed by centrifugation for 10 minutes at 25 000 x g (17 000 r.p.m.) in a No. 40 rotor of the Beckman Spinco preparative ultra-centrifuge (Model L). The supernatant was spun at 105 000 x g (34 700 r.p.m.) in the No. 50 rotor for

45 minutes. The resultant reddish-brown pellet was taken up into 2 ml of the sucrose solution, gently homogenised, the protein concentration determined, and stored on solid CO_2.

The particles were termed SP_{HL} by Sanadi, who found them to be actively phosphorylating. However, we found that the particles were not phosphorylating, and therefore called them ETP.

<u>NADH-CoQ reductase.</u>

The ETP was thawed and diluted to a protein concentration of 8 mg/ml. Phosphate buffer 1M pH 6,8 was added to a final concentration of 10mM and the pH adjusted to 6,8. The suspension was centrifuged for 15 minutes at 39 000 x g (22 000 r.p.m.) in a No. 50 rotor of the Beckman Spinco centrifuge. The pellet which was deposited, was suspended in double distilled, deionised water to a protein concentration of 25 mg/ml. The mixture was then homogenised, the pH adjusted to 5,3 with acetic acid 1M, and redistilled ethanol 95% v/v added to 11% of the particulate volume. The suspension was placed in a waterbath at 45°C, so that the temperature within the vessel containing the preparation was kept at 43°C for 15 minutes with continuous agitation.

The extract was cooled to 10°C, neutralised with

0,5M .../

0,5M NaOH, and centrifuged for 30 minutes at 39 000 x g (22 000 r.p.m.) in the Beckman No. 50 rotor. The alcoholic supernatant which contained NADH-CoQ reductase, was decanted and kept on ice. The protein concentration was determined, and the preparation gave reproduceable results for one week.

Protein determination by a biuret method.

(Gornall *et al* 1949)

Biuret Reagent: 1,50 gms cupric sulfate + 6,0 gms Na-K-Tartrate were dissolved in 500 ml water. 300 ml NaOH 10% (w/v) was added and diluted to one litre.

Reagents	Blank	Standard			Unknown
	ml	protein 8 mg/ml	protein 4 mg/ml	protein 2 mg/ml	ml
Mitochondrial suspension	-	-	-	-	0,1
5% deoxycholate	-	-	-	-	0,2
Water (d.d.)	1,0	0,8	0,9	0,95	0,7
Standard: Albumin 40 mg/ml.	-	0,2	0,1	0,05	-
Total Volume	1,0	1,0	1,0	1,0	1,0
	Left standing for 5 minutes.				
Biuret Reagent	4,0	4,0	4,0	4,0	4,0

Shaken, left at room temp. for 45 minutes and the O.D. measured at 540 nm.

Oxygen Uptake.

Oxygen uptake, by either mitochondria or ETP, was measured at 30^{0}C. with a Clarke-type electrode (YSI Model 53 Oxygen Monitor, Yellow Springs Instrument Company, Ohio). For inhibition studies, the µl quantities of halothane employed were drawn off from 0,1M and 1M solutions of halothane in ethanol.

1. NADH-linked substrates:

The basal incubation medium had the following constituents, in the given concentrations: KCl 50mM, tris 25mM, $MgCl_2$ 8mM, sucrose 100mM and pH 7,5 (modification of Ernster et al 1962). Inorganic phosphate (Pi) was added (from stock K_2HPO_4 1M, pH 7,5) to a final concentration of 10mM. The total volume of the incubation medium was 2,5 ml; the concentration of HBHM 1 mg protein/ml.

Oxygen uptake was measured in the presence of substrate (state I), 10mM Pi (State II) and 0,4mM ADP (State III).

Oxidation coupled to sites I, II and III of phosphorylation was measured in the presence of 2-oxoglutarate, glutamate, pyruvate plus malate, all at final concentrations of 10mM.

Oxidation coupled to site III was measured in the presence of N. N. N'. N'. tetra methyl-p-phenylenediamine (TMPD) - coupled non-enzymically from added ascorbate (10mM).

2. NADH-oxidase was assayed according to Minakami _et al_ (1964) and King (1967).

The incubation medium (final volume 2,38 ml) contained: phosphate 100mM, pH 7,8, Cyt.c. 0,03mM, ETP or HBHM 800 µgms; NADH 0,43 mM was added to start the reaction.

3. Succinate oxidase (King 1967).

The incubation medium (final volume 2,7ml) contained: phosphate buffer 111mM, pH 7,8, Cyt.c. 0,04mM, ETP or HBHM 800 µgms; succinate 10mM was added to start the reaction.

Calculation.

Oxygen uptake was calculated according to the following equation:

oxygen uptake µatoms / minute / mg. protein =

$$\left[\frac{\text{Units/min.}}{X_{100}} \times O_{2X_{100}} \times 2 \times V\right] \times 1/m \text{ mg.}$$

where Units/min. = the slope of the curve read from the recorder chart paper, which was marked 0 to 100 units.

X_{100} = X - Y where X is the pen deflection when the electrode was equilibrated with air-saturated buffer.

Y is the pen deflection when oxygen tension in the buffer = 0mm Hg (anaerobic).

Oxygen concentration (X_{100}) in the medium at 30°C. is taken as 235 µmoles / L.

$\therefore$ µatoms O_2/ml = 0,235 x 2 = 0,470

V = volume of the incubation medium.

m = mgms protein / total volume of mitochondrial suspension.

Enzymic Assays.

All assays were performed at 30°C. in a Zeiss PMQ II spectrophotometer, using microcuvettes, in which the total volume was 0,6 ml. *Solutions were preincubated in microcells for 2.6 mins. prior to addition of particles to start the reaction.* When ETP was under investigation, KCN was added to a final concentration of 1mM. Solutions of NADH were prepared and used within 4 hours. Halothane was withdrawn from 0,1M and 1,0M solutions as required, *prior to addition of particles.* Methods used are those of Pharo <u>et al</u> (1966) and Sanadi <u>et al</u> (1967).

1. NADH-Ubiquinone (CoQ or Menadione) reductase was measured in terms of NADH oxidation and change in O.D. at 340 nm. The assay mixture contained tris sulfate 50mM pH 8,0, Menadione 0,14mM, (0,07mM CoQ_6 or CoQ_{10}), NADH 0,13mM, ETP protein 160 µg/ml.
Menadione and CoQ_6 were dissolved in methanol, CoQ_{10} in ethanol.

2. NADH-ferricyanide reductase was assayed by following the reduction of ferricyanide by NADH as a change in O.D. at 410 nm. The reaction mixture contained tris-sulfate 50mM pH 7,5, potassium ferricyanide 1,3mM and NADH 0,4mM, ETP protein 8µg/ml.

3. NADH-Cyt.c. reductase was assayed by following Cyt.c. reduction spectrophotometrically at 550 nm. The assay mixture contained tris-sulfate 50mM pH 8,5, Cyt.c. 0,1mM and NADH 0,13mM, ETP protein 8µg/ml. *Slit width 0,03.*

Calculations .../

Calculations.

Calculations of the results from these assays involved the following equations as required:

(i) Rate of reaction: The tangent was drawn to the slope of the curve of O.D. vs t(time) at 0,25 seconds. Values of O.D. were extrapolated to 1 and 0 minutes. Therefore, Rate/min = $O.D._{(1'-0')}$ x 4 (arbitrary units.)

(ii) Units/min = Rate/min - Nonenzymatic rate.

(iii) Rate/mgm protein: $\frac{\text{Units/min}}{\text{mgms protein in volume of extract used.}}$

(iv) Relative Activity = x/y x 100%

where y = Units/min when there is no inhibitor.

where x = Units/min when inhibitor is present.

(v) Activity/ml : $\frac{\text{Units/min}}{\text{Vol. of extract used}}$.

Polarigraphic Determinations on HBHM and Submitochondrial Particles.

The respiration of whole mitochondria was studied initially using succinate or an NADH-linked substrate, either glutamate, α-ketoglutarate or pyruvate + malate. Since glutamate and pyruvate + malate gave the best respiratory control and oxygen uptake, these substrates were employed as an index of NADH-linked substrate oxidation in further studies. The oxygen consumption curves in State III NADH-coupled respiration (Figs. 8 & 9) reflected an immediate inhibitive response to the addition of halothane, which was observed with a final halothane concentration in the incubation medium as low as 0,8 mM. Higher concentrations of halothane (4,0mM and above) could almost completely inhibit pyruvate + malate-supported respiration. At comparable concentrations of succinate (Fig. 10) oxidation of this substrate was unaffected by halothane, and in some instances, slightly enhanced. Succinate (10mM) added to a pyruvate + malate medium, oxidation of which was inhibited 90% by halothane, overcame inhibition by the halogenated compound, indicating that the inhibitory site was at some point on the NADH-substrate side of the confluence of the succinate and NADH-linked pathways. Data derived from rates of utilisation of oxygen by these three substrates, as revealed by the oxygen electrode, are given in Table 2.

Table 2 .../

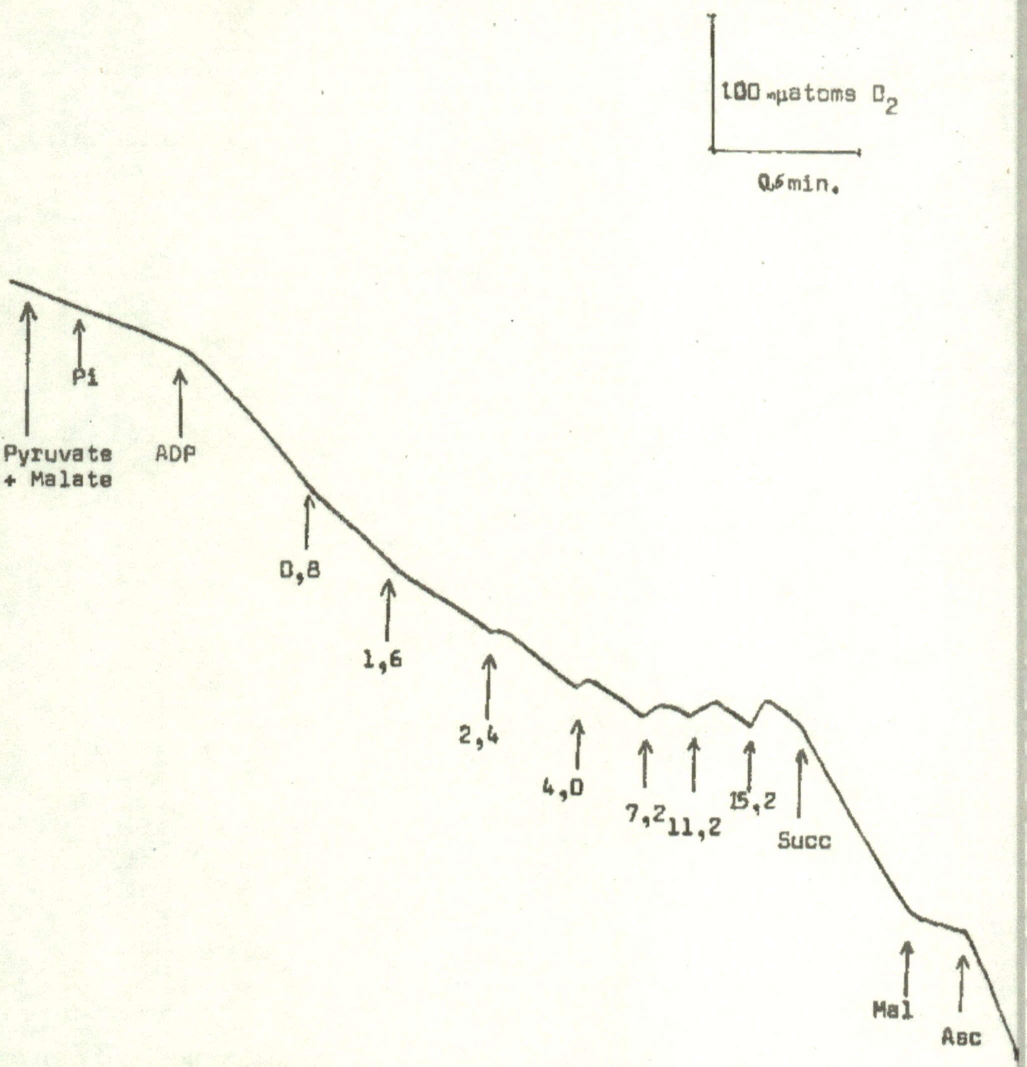

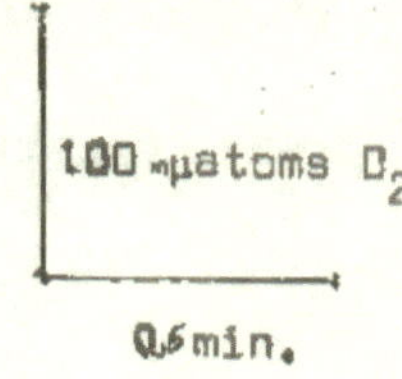

<u>Fig. 8.</u> The Effect of Halothane on the Oxidation of <u>NADH-linked substrates of HBHM:</u>

Incubation medium as described in the text, with pyruvate + malate (10 mM) as substrate.

The figures below the arrow indicate final concentrations (mM) of halothane present in the reaction mixture. Pi (10 mM), ADP (2 mM), Succ (Succinate 10 mM), Mal (Malonate 10 mM) and Asc (Ascorbate 10 mM) were added as indicated.

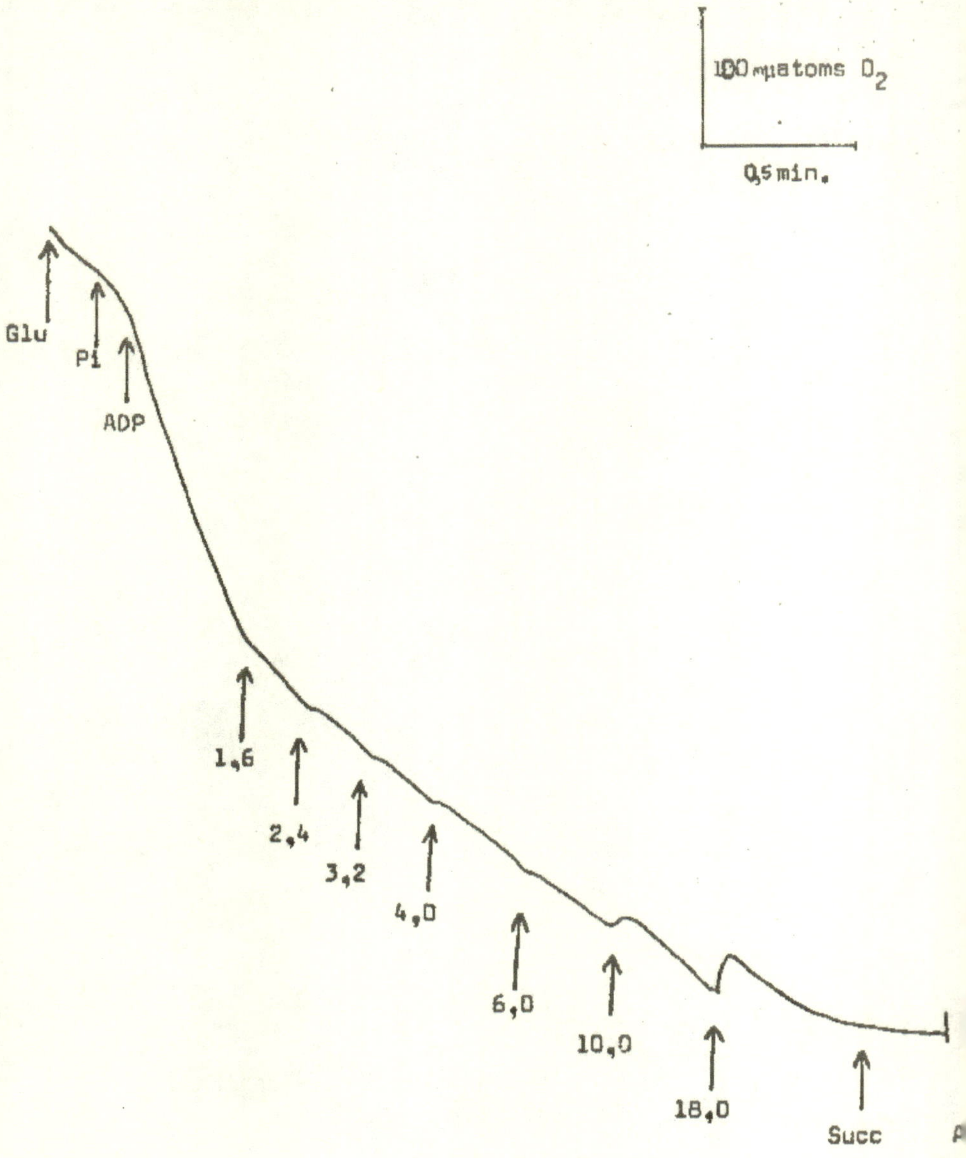

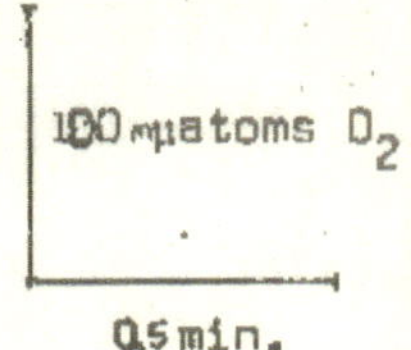

<u>Fig. 9</u> The effect of Halothane on the Oxidation of NADH-linked Substrates of HāHM.

With glutamate (10 mM) as substrate. Final halothane concentrations (mM) are given below the arrows. Pi (10 mM), ADP (1 mM), Succ (Succinate 10 mM) and Asc (Ascorbate 10 mM) were added as indicated.

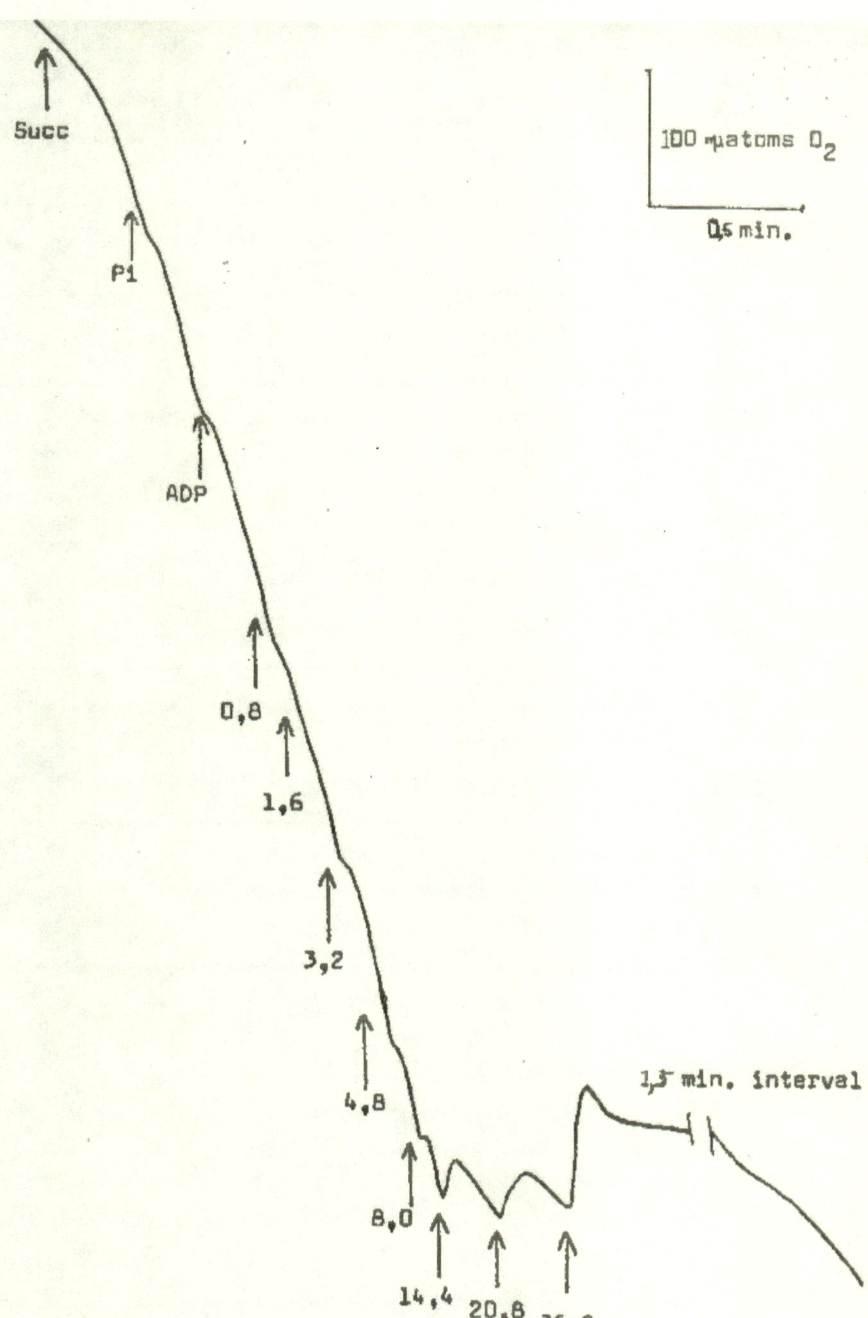

Fig. 10. The effect of halothane on succinate oxidation of HBHM with succinate (10mM) as substrate. Figures below the arrows represent final halothane concentration (mM) in the reaction mixture Pi (10mM) and ADP (1mM) were added as indicated.

Table 2. The effects of Halothane on the Oxygen Consumption of whole HBHM.

Halothane	Succinate		Glutamate		Pyruvate + Malate	
mM	O_2 Uptake	% Inhibition.	O_2 Uptake	% Inhibition.	O_2 Uptake	% Inhibition.
-	0,199	0	0,124	0	0,067	0
0,8	0,195	2	-	-	0,064	5
1,6	0,189	5	0,075	39	0,039	42
3,2	0,184	8	0,045	63	0,038	44
8,0	0,175	10	0,043	65	0,032	53

Oxygen uptake: µatoms of oxygen utilised. minute $^{-1}$mg protein^{-1}

Table 3. The Effect of Halothane on NADH Oxidase Activity of HBHM.

Halothane mM	O_2 Uptake	% Inhibition
-	0,620	0
1,26	0,175	72
2,10	0,127	79
2,50	0,101	84
3,80	0,051	92
5,00	0,031	95

Oxygen uptake: µatoms of oxygen utilised. minute $^{-1}$mg protein^{-1}.

Table 3 .../

Table 3 presents comparable information on the effect of halothane on HBHM respiration when NADH was substrate. As seen from the high rate of oxygen consumption, NADH was readily oxidised by the preparation. Inhibition by halothane followed a similar course, but was more marked than that of NADH-linked substrates (Tables 2 and 3). Whereas oxidation of NADH or NADH-linked substrates was in each instance readily susceptible to inhibition by halothane, succinate oxidation was relatively insensitive.

Oxidation by submitochondrial particles (ETP), which are nonphosphorylating was more sensitive to inhibition by halothane than were HBHM. (Figs. 11, 12, and 13). The magnitude of the difference in the effect of halothane on oxidation of the two substrates, NADH and succinate, is more apparent, because, at concentrations between 0,6 and 8,0mM of halothane, succinoxidase was actually stimulated.

Approximately 16 times the concentration of halothane is required to inhibit oxidation of succinate by ETP to the same extent as for NADH-linked processes. (Table 4).

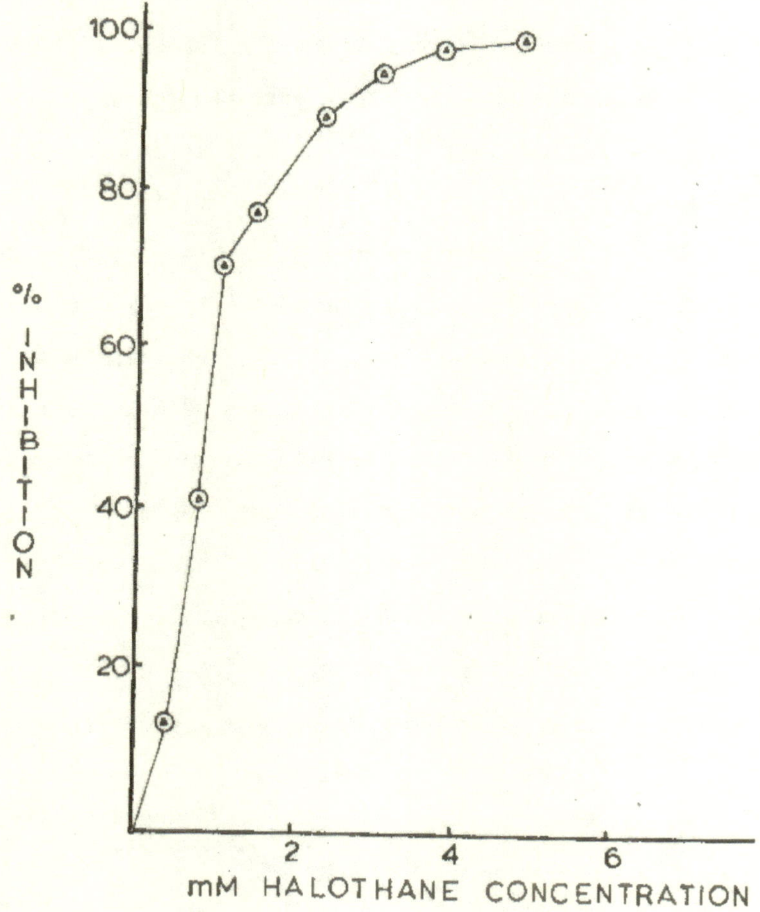

Fig.11: ETP: NADH OXIDASE INHIBITION BY HALOTHANE

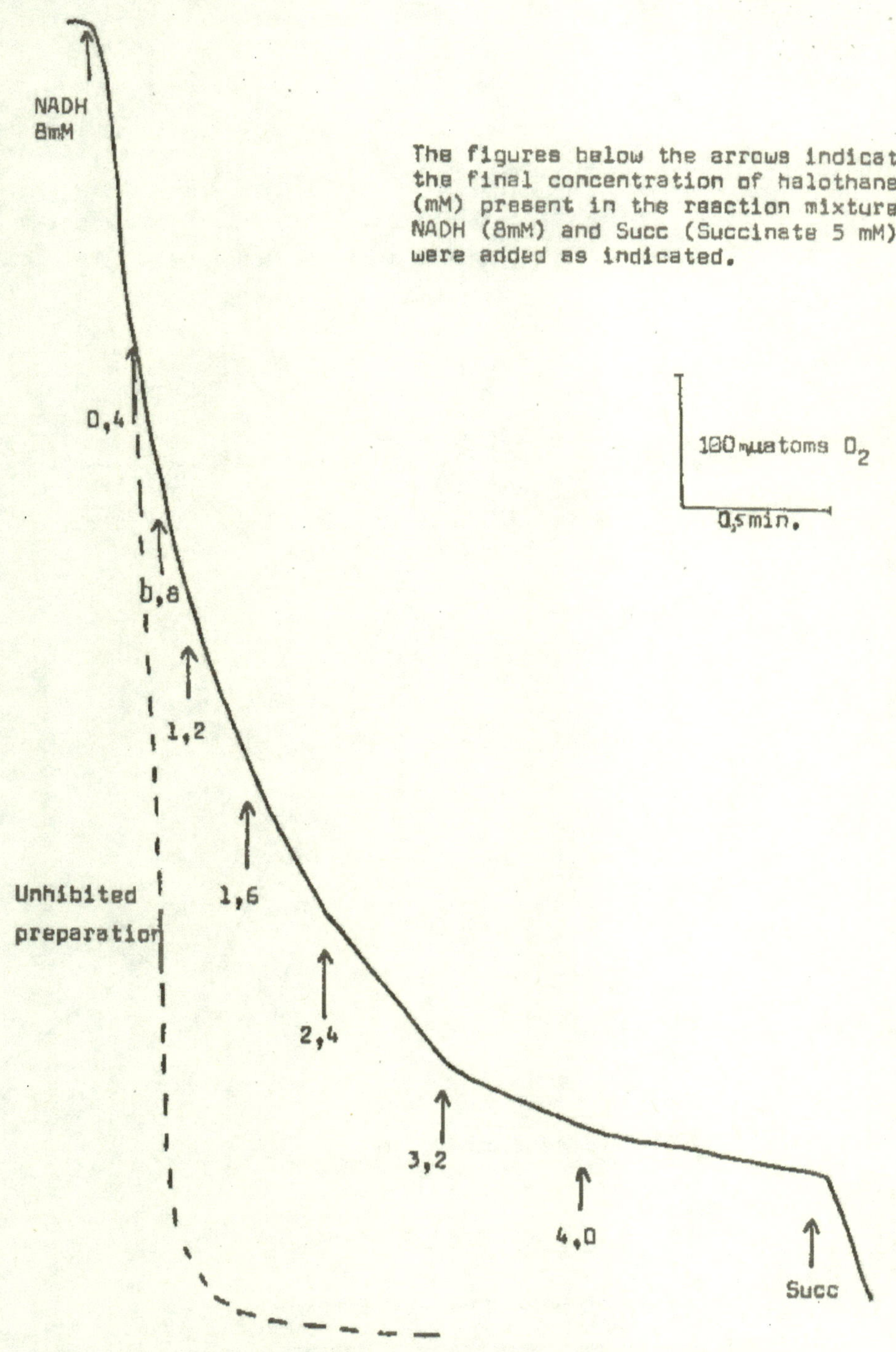

Fig. 12: Halothane Inhibition of NADH Oxidase Activity of ETP.

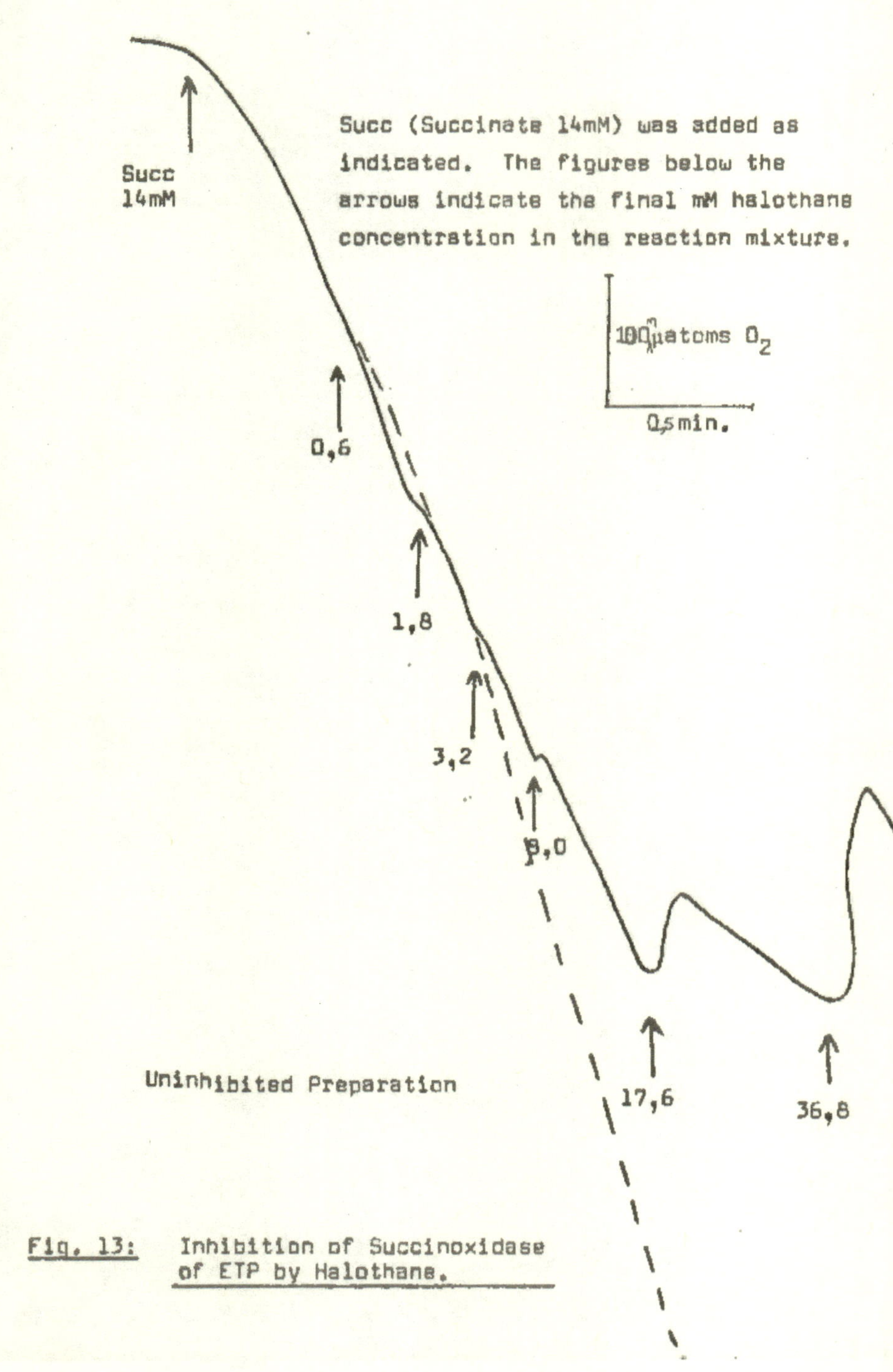

Fig. 13: Inhibition of Succinoxidase of ETP by Halothane.

Table 4. The Effect of Halothane upon Oxidase Activity of ETP.

NADH Oxidase			Succinoxidase		
Halothane mM	O_2 Uptake	% Inhibition	Halothane mM	O_2 Uptake	% Inhibition.
-	0,580	0	-	0,165	0
0,4	0,503	13	0,6	0,227	-38
0,8	0,344	41	1,8	0,241	-46
1,2	0,171	71	3,2	0,241	-46
1,6	0,135	77	8,0	0,275	-67
2,5	0,065	89	17,6	0,062	62
3,2	0,036	94	36,8	0,003	98
4,0	0,020	97			
5,0	0,014	98*			

Oxygen uptake: µatoms of oxygen utilised. minute^{-1}mg protein^{-1}.

* Inhibition could not be relieved by the addition of uncouplers such as DNP (1mM) or Dicoumarol (0,4mM).

Because of their simpler nature, ETP were further studied from the viewpoint of the manner in which they are inactivated by halothane.

Table 5. The Effect of NADH concentration on Oxygen Uptake by ETP.

v	NADH mM	1/v	1/s
0,246	0,340	4,06	2,90
0,417	0,680	2,40	1,50
0,649	1,360	1,54	0,70
0,885	2,720	1,13	0,40

v : µatoms of oxygen utilised. minute^{-1}mg protein^{-1}.

s : substrate concentration (NADH mM).

The relationship between NADH concentration and the rate of oxygen uptake in ETP was first investigated, (Table 5) and was found to conform to typical Michaelis Menton kinetics (Fig. 14). A Lineweaver-Burk double reciprocal plot (Fig. 15 , Table 5) gave a straight line, from which maximum velocity, calculated from the intercept on the y axis, was 1,39 µatoms oxygen utilised. minute^{-1} mg protein^{-1}. From the slope (K_{NADH}/V) of the graph, the Michaelis constant K_{NADH} was calculated to be 1,60 mM.

A comparable experiment to determine the effect of halothane on oxygen uptake with varying concentrations of substrate (NADH) was made. Halothane was present in concentration 0, 0,4, 0,8, 1,2, or 1,6 mM.

Table 6 .../

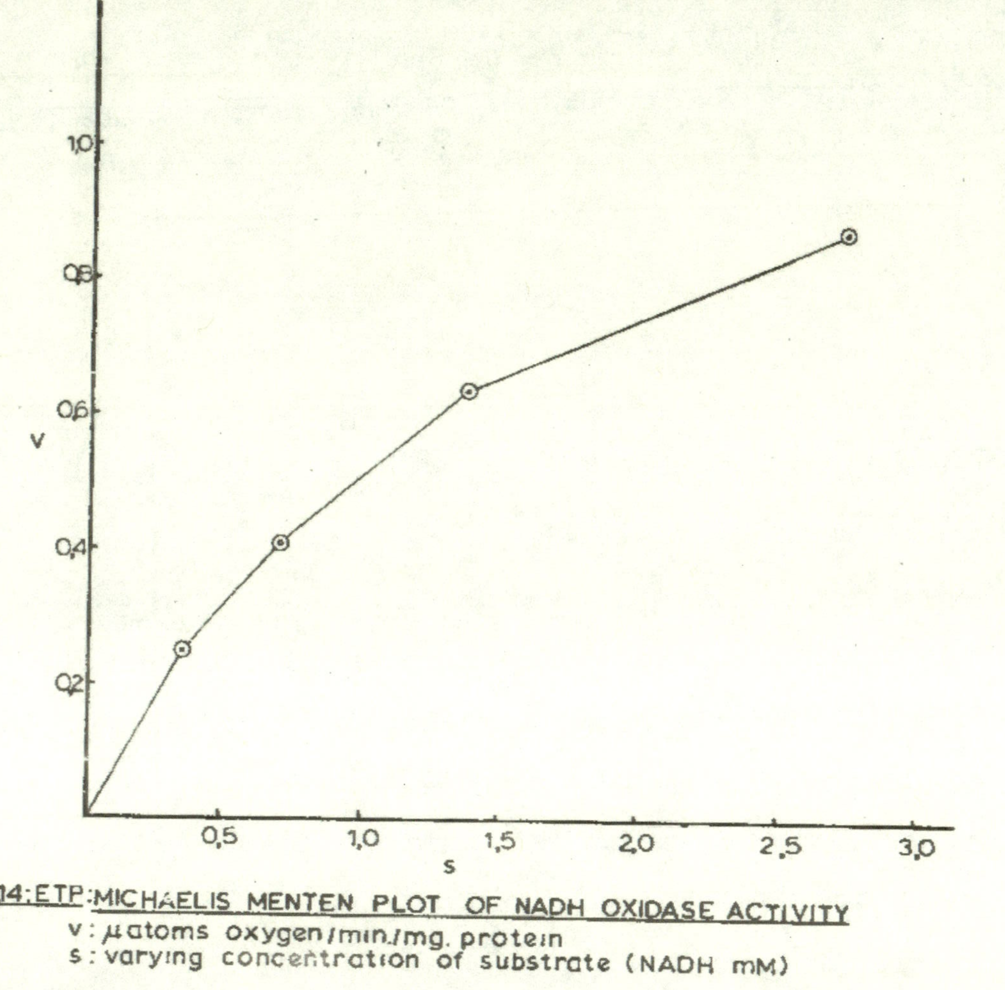

Fig14: ETP: MICHAELIS MENTEN PLOT OF NADH OXIDASE ACTIVITY

v : μatoms oxygen/min./mg. protein

s : varying concentration of substrate (NADH mM)

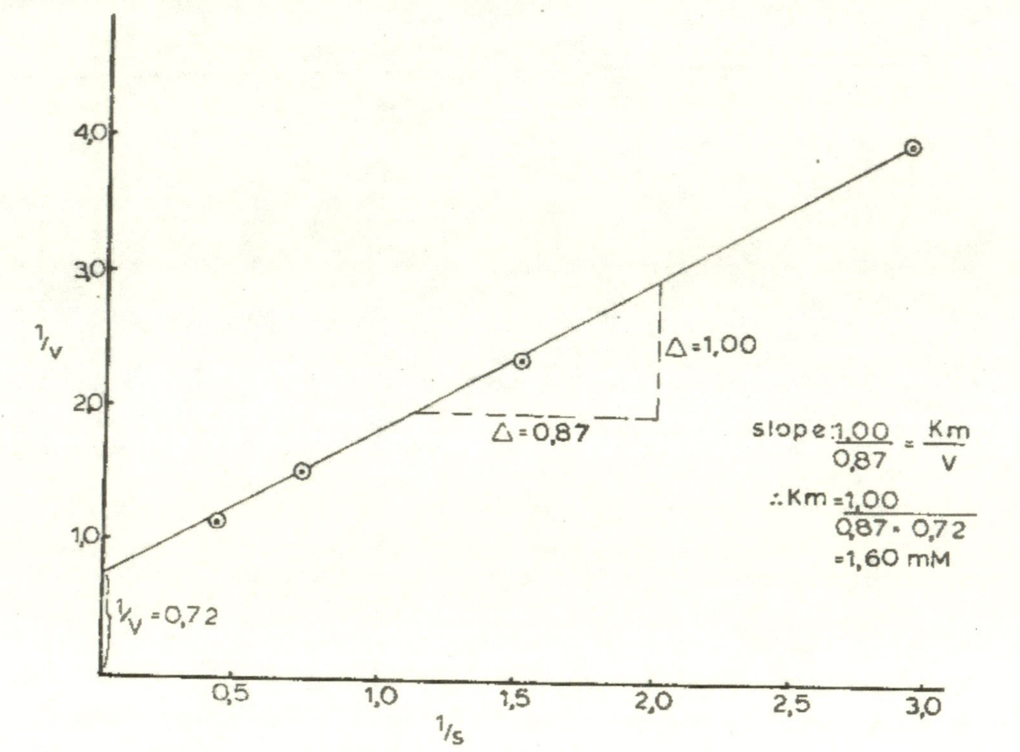

Fig.15: ETP: LINEWEAVER BURK PLOT OF NADH OXIDASE ACTIVITY

v : μ atoms oxygen/min/mg. protein

s : varying concentration of substrate (NADH mM)

Table 6. Kinetic Parameters of NADH Oxidase in ETP, in the Presence of Differing Concentrations of Halothane.

Halothane mM	1/v					1/s				
-	7,88	4,06	2,40	1,54	1,13	6,3	2,9	1,5	0,7	0,4
0,4	11,20	6,40	5,40	4,60	-	6,3	3,1	2,1	1,6	-
0,8	14,50	10,50	8,10	7,50	-	6,3	3,1	2,1	1,6	-
1,6	16,90	12,50	11,50	10,60	-	6,3	3,1	2,1	1,6	-
1,2	16,30	10,70	9,40	8,10	-	6,3	3,1	2,1	1,6	-

Each value in the Table is the mean of 3 - 4 determinations.

v : µatoms oxygen utilised. minute $^{-1}$ mg protein^{-1}.

s : NADH concentration expressed in mM.

Reciprocals of velocity and substrate concentration were plotted for each concentration of halothane, and these were linearly related, straight lines with equal slopes (Fig. 16), and V maximum decreased accordingly. Intercepts of these lines on the y axis increased with halothane concentration. The lines of the Lineweaver-Burk plots are parallel, and of the pattern associated with uncompetitive inhibition (Cleland 1963). K_{NADH} was determined from the slope (K_{NADH}/V) at different halothane concentrations. The results presented in Table 7 show that K_{NADH} falls with rising concentration of halothane, i.e. with progressive inhibition of NADH

oxidase .../

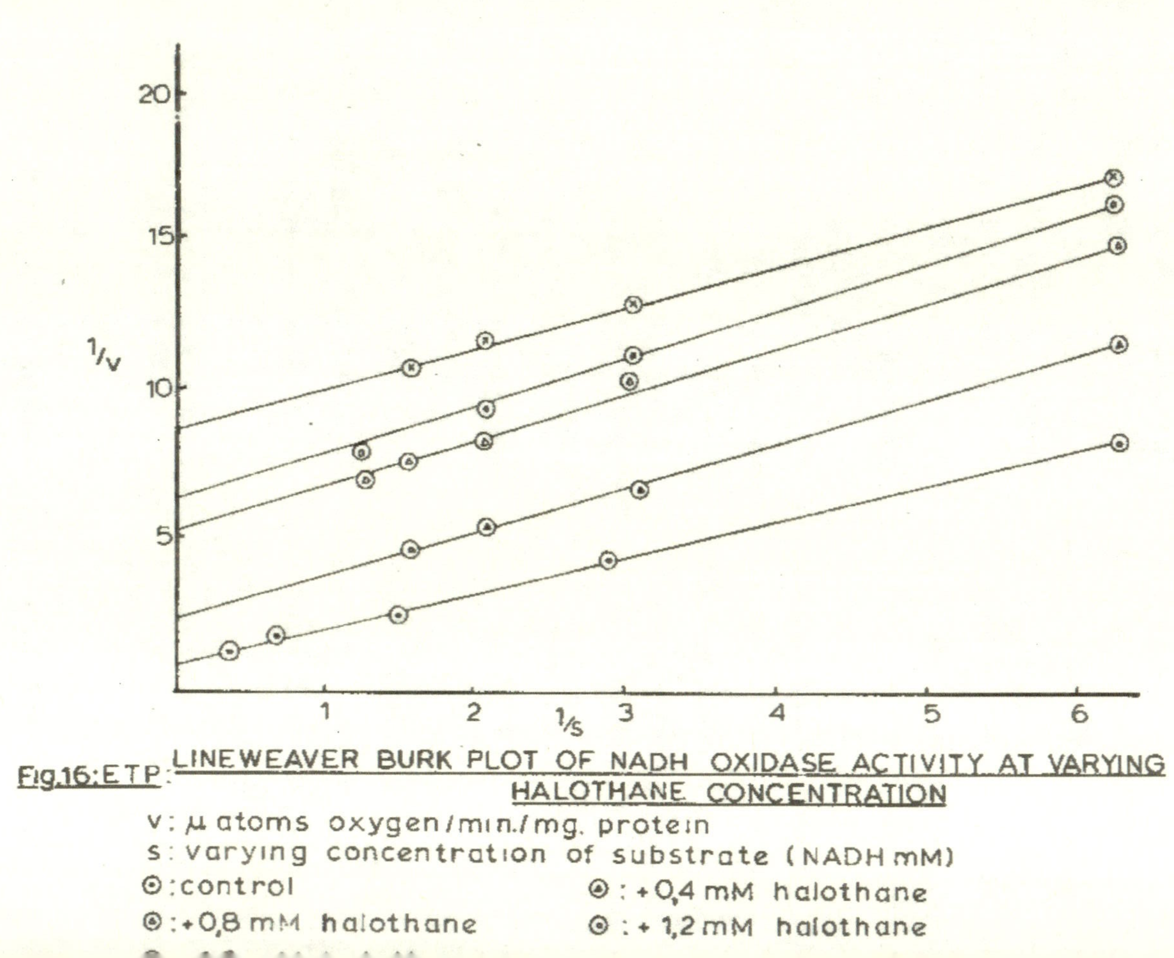

Fig.16:ETP: LINEWEAVER BURK PLOT OF NADH OXIDASE ACTIVITY AT VARYING HALOTHANE CONCENTRATION

v: μ atoms oxygen/min./mg. protein
s: varying concentration of substrate (NADH mM)
⊙: control ⊙: + 0,4 mM halothane
⊙: + 0,8 mM halothane ⊙: + 1,2 mM halothane

oxidase. (Fig. 16.)

Table 7. The Effect of Halothane on K_{NADH} of NADH Oxidase of ETP.

Halothane mM	K_{NADH} (mM)
0,0	1,60
0,4	0,64
0,8	0,29
1,2	0,25
1,6	0,16

In a separate experiment, which was similar in detail to the one just described, an attempt was made to examine the effect of different concentrations of inhibitor on the velocity of NADH oxidase at constant initial NADH concentration. The results of such a study are shown in Table 8.

Table 8 .../

Table 8. The Influence of Halothane, in Different Concentrations, on the Velocity of NAD.' Oxidation in ETP.

i	v	1/v	v_i	$1/v_i$	v/v_i	1/s
0,42	0,66	1,52	0,51	1,98	1,30	0,12
0,84	0,65	1,54	0,25	4,00	2,60	0,12
1,30	0,48	2,08	0,13	7,81	3,77	0,12
1,68	0,55	1,82	0,08	13,20	7,20	0,12
2,10	0,71	1,39	0,05	18,50	13,39	0,12

v : µatoms oxygen utilised. $minute^{-1}$.mg. $protein^{-1}$.

v_i : µatoms oxygen utilised. $minute^{-1}$.mg. $protein^{-1}$, in the presence of inhibitor.

i : concentration of inhibitor (Halothane mM).

s : NADH 8,5 mM.

A plot of V_{max} at various inhibitor concentration obtained from the Lineweaver-Burk plots shown in Fig.16, against inhibitor concentration (i) showed a straight line relationship (Table 8a, Fig.17) and is additional evidence for uncompetitive-type inhibition. The intercept on the x axis, $-K_i$, gave a value of K_i of 0,14mM.

Table 8a ..../

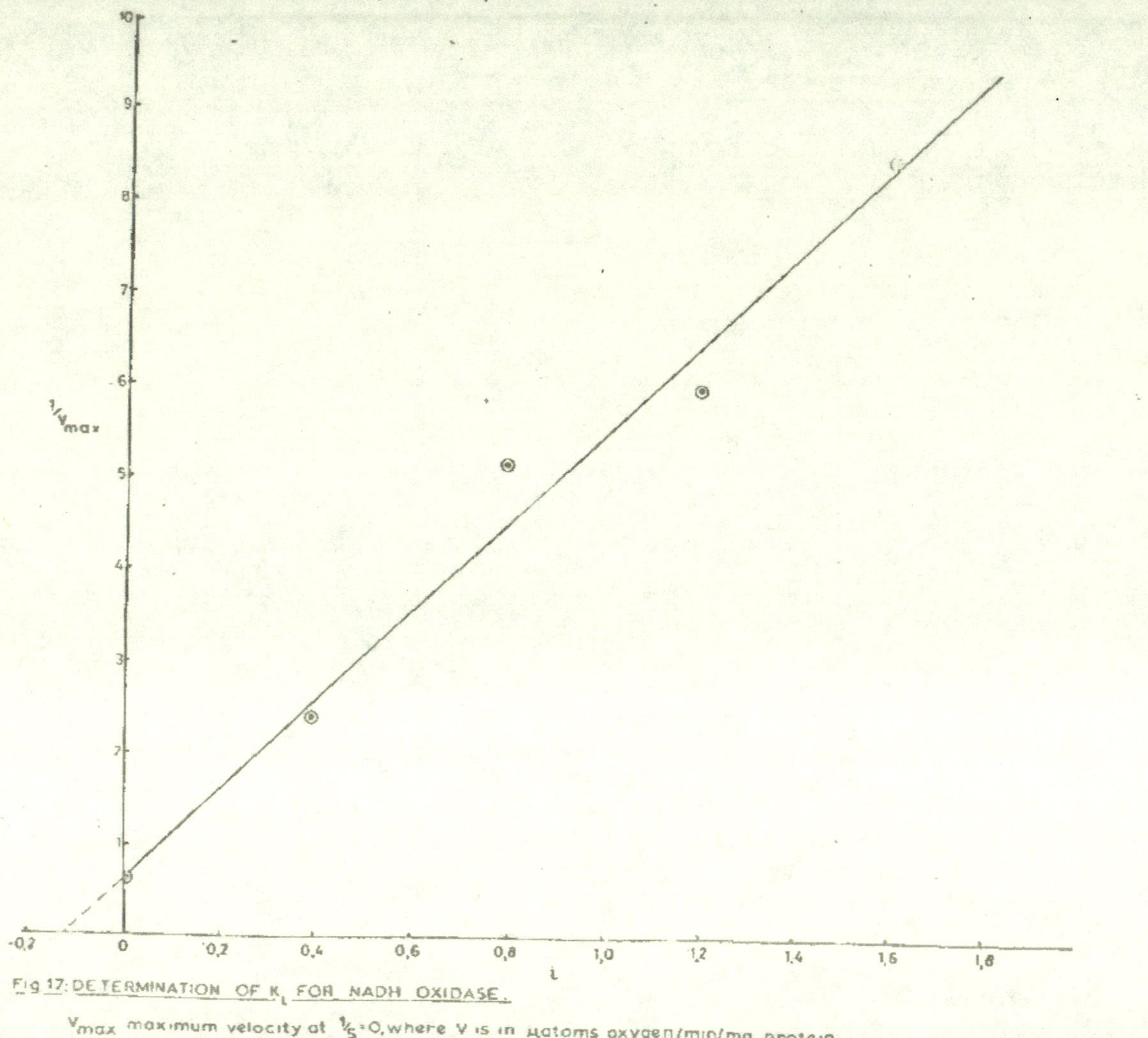

Fig 17: DETERMINATION OF K_i FOR NADH OXIDASE.

V_{max} maximum velocity at $1/S = 0$, where V is in µatoms oxygen/min/mg protein

i mM halothane

Table 8a. The Determination of K_i for NADH Oxidase.

i	V_{max}
0,0	0,63
0,4	2,40
0,8	5,15
1,2	5,97
1,6	8,47

i : concentration of inhibitor (Halothane mM).

V_{max} : maximum velocity in μatoms oxygen utilised. minute^{-1}. mg protein^{-1}.

Reversibility of Halothane Inhibition.

A suspension of ETP (or HBHM) was exposed to various concentrations of halothane in the incubation medium as before, for 5 minutes, during which time oxygen uptake was measured in the presence of 8,6 mM NADH. At the end of this period, the oxygen concentration approached zero. The mixture was then exposed to air, by removing the oxygen electrode holder, and was stirred continuously with a magnetic stirrer. After 5 minutes the electrode was replaced, 8,5 mM NADH added and the rate of oxygen utilisation again measured.

Table 9 ..../

Table 9. Reversibility of Inhibition by Halothane of NADH Oxidase.

Halothane mM	Initial Activity.		Activity After Aeration.		Activity After Evacuation.	
	O_2 Uptake	% Activity.	O_2 Uptake	% Activity.	O_2 Uptake	% Activity.
0	0,795	100	-	-	0,453	57
0,84	0,461	58	0,898	113	0,334	42
1,26	0,246	31	0,231	29	0,199	25
1,68	0,159	20	0,215	27	0,175	22
2,10	0,080	10	0,143	18	0,119	15
2,52	0,056	7	0,207	26	0,127	16
3,36	0,05	7	0,217	27	0,223	28

O_2 uptake : µatoms of oxygen utilised. minute^{-1} mg. protein^{-1}.

Table 10. The Reversibility of Halothane Inhibition of NADH Oxidase in HBHM.

Halothane mM	Initial Activity.		Activity After Aeration.		Activity after Evacuation.	
	O_2 Uptake	% Activity.	O_2 Uptake	% Activity	O_2 Uptake	% Activity.
2,5	0,052	16	0,075	23	0,106	33
3,8	0,026	8	0,046	14	0,060	19
5,0	0,016	5	0,044	14	0,057	18

O_2 uptake: µatoms of oxygen utilised. minute^{-1} mg. protein^{-1}.

Finally .../

Finally the incubation mixture was exposed to a vacuum line (± 50 mm Hg) with continuous shaking, for 5 minutes, NADH (8,5mM) added and oxygen uptake recorded as before. Data are presented in Tables 9 and 10.

The 42% inhibition induced by 0,84mM halothane was dispelled by exposure to air, indeed, a slight stimulation was noted when compared to control preparations. At higher concentrations of halothane, inhibition was only slightly abolished. After evacuation, the results were more variable and no relief of inhibition occurred, except at higher concentrations of the inhibitor. Inhibition of HBHM was studied on exposure to concentrations of halothane. A pattern of irreversibility was remarked similar to that in ETP at these concentrations. An ETP preparation, in the absence of halothane, lost 43% of its NADH oxidase activity simply following evacuation. It is, therefore, suggested that unrelieved inhibition in these experiments is a consequence of denaturation of the enzyme during frothing, which invariably occurs. Inhibition of NADH oxidation by halothane appears, therefore, to be completely reversible at low concentrations and irreversible above 2 mM. The efficiency of aeration and vacuum treatment have been confirmed by gas chromatography, which has shown that the halothane concentration in the incubation medium is lowered to undetectable levels (Berman 1969).

Table 11. .../

Table 11. The Effect of NADH on NADH Oxidase Activity of ETP.

Halothane mM	Halothane + NADH		Halothane only	
	O_2 Uptake	% Activity	O_2 Uptake	% Activity
1,16	0,115	23	0,051	10
2,0	0,112	22	0,050	10
3,2	0,060	12	0,045	9
4,6	0,049	10	0,020	4
6,0	0,013	3	0,017	3

Oxygen uptake: µatoms oxygen utilised. minute^{-1} mg. protein^{-1}.
Preincubation time : 3 minutes.

An attempt was made to determine the effect, if any, of the redox state of the mitochondrial chain on its susceptibility to inhibition by halothane. Suspensions of the mitochondrial particles (ETP) were incubated, as previously described, with various concentrations of halothane in the presence or absence of NADH (8,5 mM). After 3 minutes at 30°C in a closed chamber, NADH (8,5mM) was added to both preparations and oxygen consumption measured. The results (Table 11 and Fig. 18.) show that the inhibition by halothane was significantly less when incubated in the presence of NADH at concentrations between 1,6 and 4,6 mM.

The .../

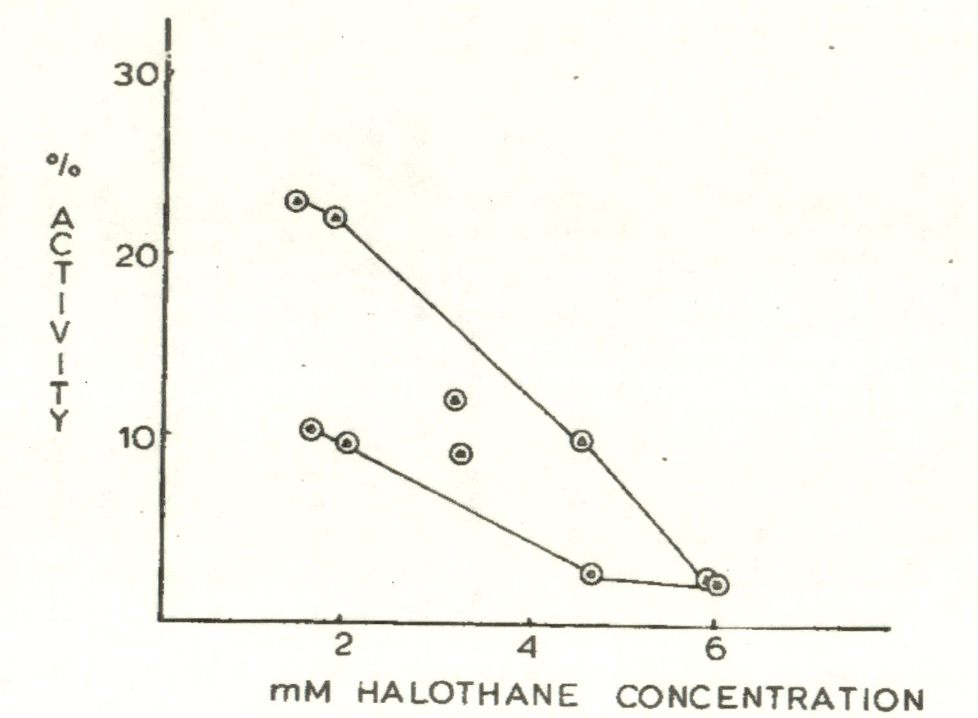

Fig18:ETP:PROTECTIVE EFFECT OF NADH ON NADH OXIDASE
⊙: preincubation with NADH
⊙: preincubation with NADH + Halothane

The preparation was inhibited by more than 95% by 6mM halothane, and at this low level of activity NADH afforded no protection.

Table 12 shows the consequence of incubating ETP alone, halothane and ETP together, with subsequent exposure of the preparation to air for 5 minutes. In this way, the possible significance of duration of contact between ETP and halothane could be evaluated. ETP were incubated, in the absence of NADH, for 10 minutes with 1,26mM halothane. A control preparation was incubated without halothane. NADH (8,5mM) was then added to the control and to the halothane-treated suspension and NADH oxidase activity assayed. Next, halothane was added to the control suspension and its effect noted. After exposure to air for 5 minutes and subsequent addition of NADH (8,5mM), NADH oxidase activity was again measured. It transpired (Table 12) that incubation of ETP with halothane for 10 minutes caused only a slightly greater inhibition (68%) of NADH oxidase than the inhibition incurred (63%) when halothane was added later. Exposure to air proved that inhibition in both preparations could be partially reversed and that the reversal was slightly greater with the control preparation initially incubated. These results suggest that the duration of contact without halothane of enzyme and inhibitor has only a slight influence on the magnitude of inhibition, and on its reversibility.

Table 12. .../

Table 12. The Effect of Halothane when Incubated with ETP.

Halothane mM	ETP Alone		ETP + Halothane (1,26mM)	
	O_2Uptake	% Activity	O_2Uptake	% Activity
-	0,584	100		
1,26	0,218	37	0,184	32
*	0,403*	69*	0,332*	57*

* Exposure to air for 5 minutes.

Oxygen uptake: µatoms oxygen utilised. minute $^{-1}$ mg. protein^{-1}.

The Effects of Various Halogenated Hydrocarbons and of Diethyl Ether on NADH Oxidase. (Table 13 and Fig. 19).

NADH oxidase was exposed in turn to several halogenated hydrocarbons and to diethyl ether. Different volumes of a 1M solution of each inhibitor in ethanol were added to the incubation mixture, as previously described for halothane. Diethyl ether in concentrations up to 2mM had no effect on NADH oxidase, and above this level it inhibited oxygen uptake to a much lesser extent than did halogenated hydrocarbons. The halogenated compounds carbon tetrachloride, chloroform, methallyl chloride and halothane were inhibitive at low concentrations. Oxygen utilisation of preparations containing NADH in which oxidation had been inhibited to 98% or more by carbon tetrachloride, chloroform or methallyl chloride, was stimulated significantly with 8,4mM succinate. These inhibitors, therefore, act specifically on the NADH dehydrogenase complex, as does halothane.

Table 13. .../

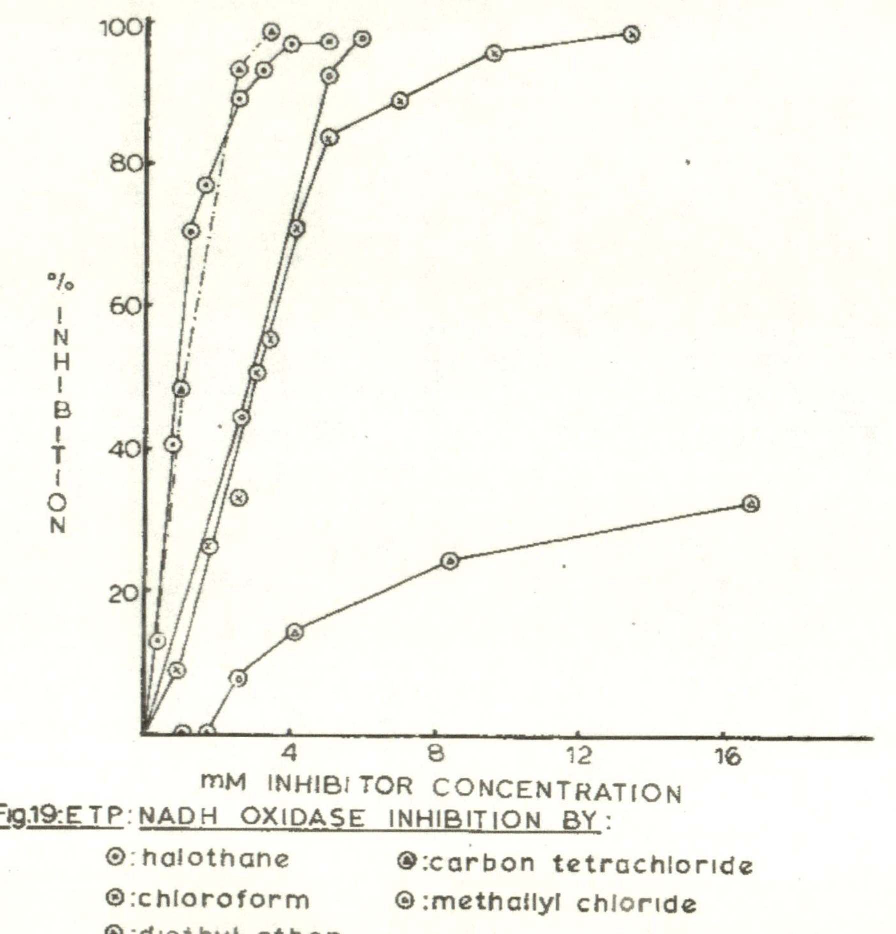

Fig.19: ETP: NADH OXIDASE INHIBITION BY:

⊙: halothane ⊗: carbon tetrachloride
⊙: chloroform ⊙: methallyl chloride
⊗: diethyl ether

Table 13. The Action of Halogenated Hydrocarbons and of Diethyl Ether on NADH Oxidase in ETP.

Halothane			Carbon Tetrachloride			Chloroform		
mM	O_2 Uptake	% Inhibition	mM	O_2 Uptake	% Inhibition	mM	O_2 Uptake	% Inhibition
-	0,580	0	-	0,493	0	-	0,354	0
0,4	0,503	13	0,84	0,252	49	0,84	0,324	9
0,8	0,344	41	2,52	0,031	94	1,68	0,259	27
1,2	0,171	71	3,36	0,006	99	2,52	0,229	35
1,6	0,135	77				2,94	0,176	50
2,5	0,065	89				3,36	0,157	57
3,2	0,036	94				4,20	0,103	71
4,0	0,020	97				5,04	0,057	84
5,0	0,014	98				7,10	0,040	87
						9,66	0,012	96
						13,40	0,006	98

Methallyl Chloride			Diethyl Ether		
mM	O_2Uptake	% Inhibition	mM	O_2Uptake	% Inhibition
-	0,504	0	-	0,384	0
0,84	0,560	-11	0,84	0,384	0
2,52	0,280	44	1,68	0,384	0
5,04	0,034	93	2,52	0,354	8
5,88	0,010	98	4,20	0,330	14
			8,40	0,291	24
			16,80	0,259	33

Oxygen uptake: µatoms oxygen utilised. minute $^{-1}$ mg. protein^{-1}.

Results .../

Results of a study of inhibitors with differing halogen content is given in Table 14. At 3mM concentration, carbon tetrachloride is the most potent inhibitor. If the degree of inhibition of NADH oxidase is plotted against the number of helogen atoms per molecule of inhibitor or activator (Fig. 20), it is immediately evident that the richness of halogenation contributes largely to the inhibitory action of these compounds. Mono- and di-chloro compounds are slightly stimulatory, but more highly halogenated substances are inhibitory. The one unsaturated compound tested, methallyl chloride, is anomalous and does not fit into the pattern.

Table 14. Inhibition of NADH Oxidase by Halogenated Hydrocarbons and by Diethyl Ether.

Inhibitor	Structure	% Inhibition.
Diethyl Ether	$(C_2H_5)_2O$	8
2-Chloroethanol	CH_2ClCH_2OH	-24
Methallyl Chloride	$CH{=}C(CH_3)CH_2Cl$	44
Dichlormethane	CH_2Cl_2	-64
Dichlorethane	$Cl(CH_2)_2Cl$	-60
Chloroform	$CHCl_3$	51
Carbon Tetrachloride	CCl_4	94
Halothane	$CF_3CHBrCl$	90

The concentration of all the compounds was 3mM.

Table .../

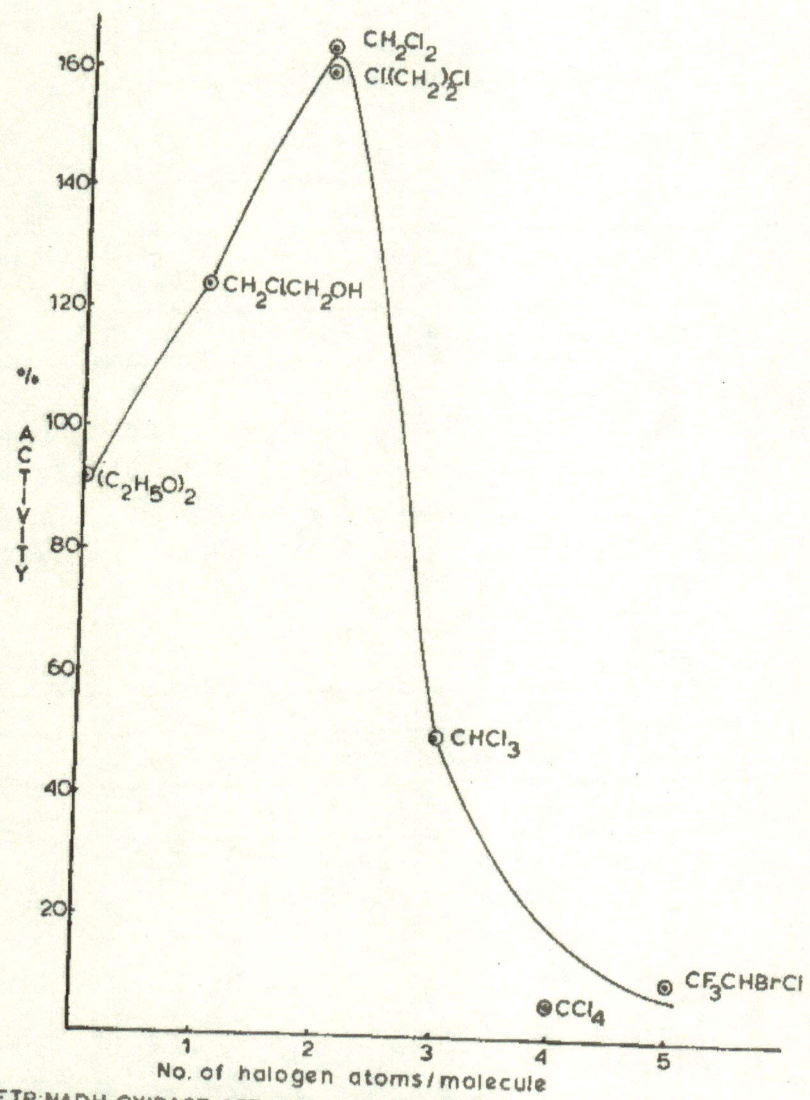

Fig.20: ETP: NADH OXIDASE ACTIVITY WITH VARIOUS INHIBITORS (3 mM)

Table 15 and Fig. 21 give the values of v/v_i of ETP NADH Oxidase accruing from various concentrations of halogens and of ether. None of the plots is strictly linear, all having an upward slope similar to that of halothane, which strengthens the evidence that this represents a complex type of inhibition, which is neither totally competitive nor non-competitive.

Table 15. Kinetics of the Action of Some Halogenated Compounds and of Diethyl Ether on NADH Oxidase.

Chloroform		Dichlor-methane		Diethyl ether		Chloro-ethanol		Dichlorethane	
mM	v/v_i	mM	v/v_i	mM	v/v_i	mM	v/v_i	mM	v/v_i
0,84	1,14	0,84	0,58	0,84	1,0	0,84	0,9	0,84	0,70
1,68	1,20	2,52	0,61	1,68	1,0	2,52	0,8	2,52	0,63
2,52	1,60	5,88	0,79	2,52	1,1	4,20	0,9	5,88	0,85
2,94	2,00	12,60	2,13	3,36	1,1	7,56	1,2	12,60	2,35
3,36	2,30			4,20	1,2			21,00	26,90
4,20	3,50			8,40	1,7				
5,04	4,40								
7,10	8,70								

Carbon Tetrachloride		Methallyl Chloride		Halothane	
mM	v/v_i	mM	v/v_i	mM	v/vi
0,84	1,96	0,84	0,90	0,42	1,30
2,52	15,90	2,52	1,80	0,84	2,60
3,36	82,20	5,04	14,82	1,30	3,77
		5,88	50,40	1,68	7,20
				2,10	13,39

v : µatoms of oxygen utilised. minute^{-1} mg. protein^{-1}.
v_i: µatoms of oxygen utilised. minute^{-1} mg. protein^{-1}.
i : inhibitor concentration (mM)

Spectrophotometric .../

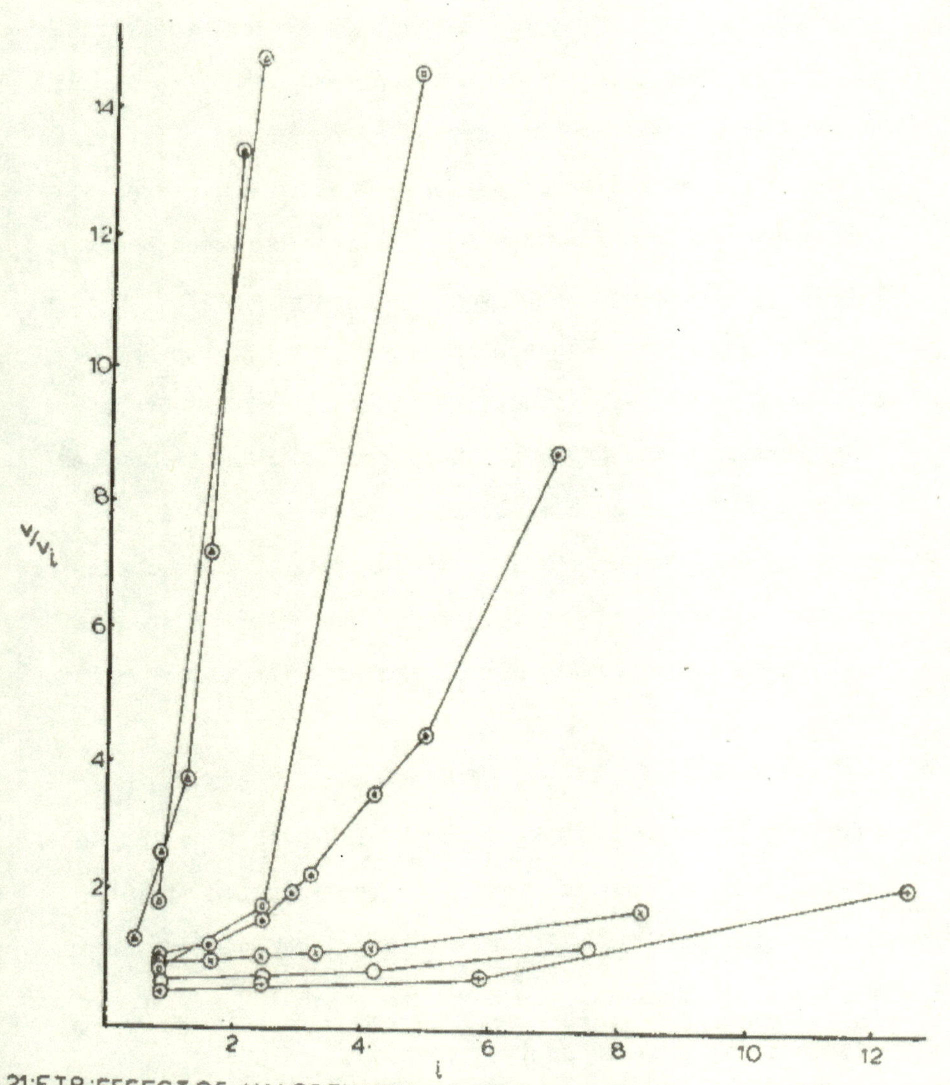

Fig.21:ETP: EFFECT OF HALOGENATED HYDROCARBONS ON NADH OXIDASE ACTIVITY

v/v_i: ratio of velocity in the presence & absence of inhibitor

i: varying concention of inhibitors (mM)

- ⓐ: halothane
- ⓑ: chloroform
- ⓒ: diethyl ether
- O: chloroethanol
- ⓓ: carbon tetrachloride
- ⓔ: methallyl chloride
- ⊕: dichlormethane

Spectrophotometric Determination of NADH Dehydrogenase.

NADH dehudrogenase was assayed by several spectrophotometric procedures which are based either on change in optical density of NADH at 340 nm, or on corresponding alterations in spectral absorption of various electron acceptors. Spectrophotometric readings were plotted on graph paper and representative examples of each assay are depicted in Figs. 22 and 23. Reactions were linear for varying periods, shortest for the higher analogue of NADH-CoQ reductase. NADH-Menadione and NADH-$K_3Fe(CN)_6$ reductases activity was maintained for up to 5 minutes. NADH-Cyt.c. reductase activity fell away rapidly after 3 minutes. These findings are similar to those observed by other workers (Sanadi 1967).

Enzyme velocity was calculated from the linear portions of the curve.

The specific activity of NADH-CoQ_6 reductase and of NADH-CoQ_{10} reductase is known to be influenced by the concentration of enzymatic protein in the reaction mixture (Sanadi et al 1967). In an experiment designed to verify this, maximum activity was observed using 160μgms of mitochondrial protein in the reaction. Higher concentrations of protein were less active (Fig. 24), the reason for which is not evident, but may have something to

do .../

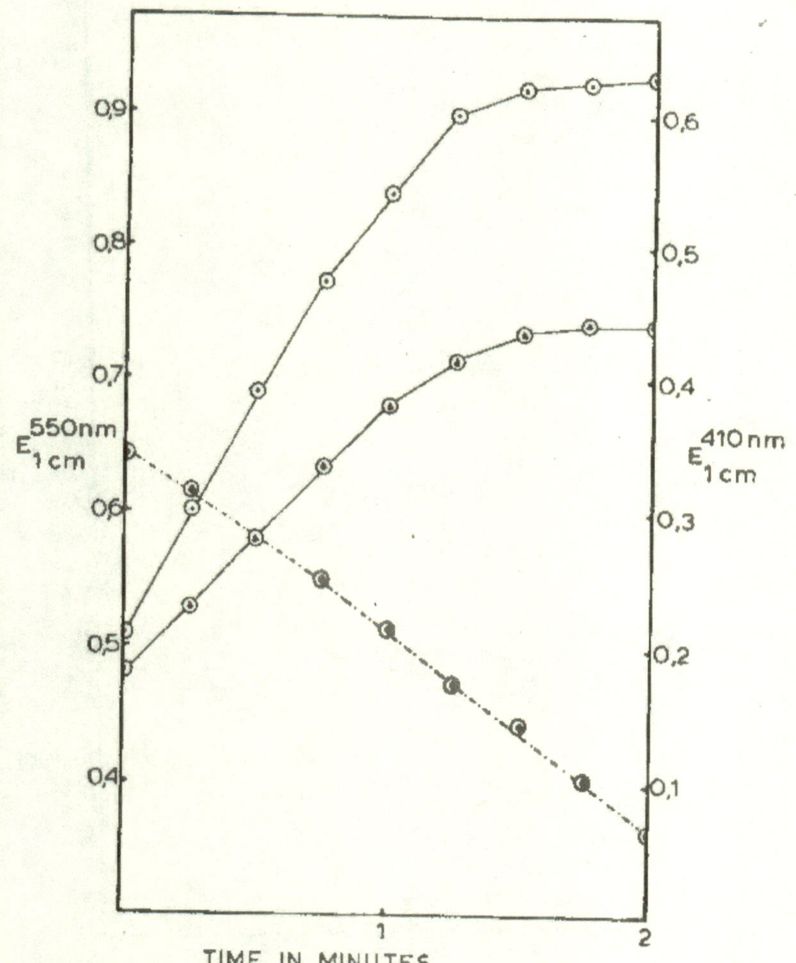

Fig.22:ETP: SPECTROPHOTOMETRIC ASSAY CURVES OF NADH-CYT.C. AND NADH-$K_3Fe(CN)_6$ REDUCTASE ACTIVITIES

⊙ : NADH-cyt.c. reductase
◎ : NADH-cyt.c. reductase + 1mM halothane
● : NADH-$K_3Fe(CN)_6$ reductase

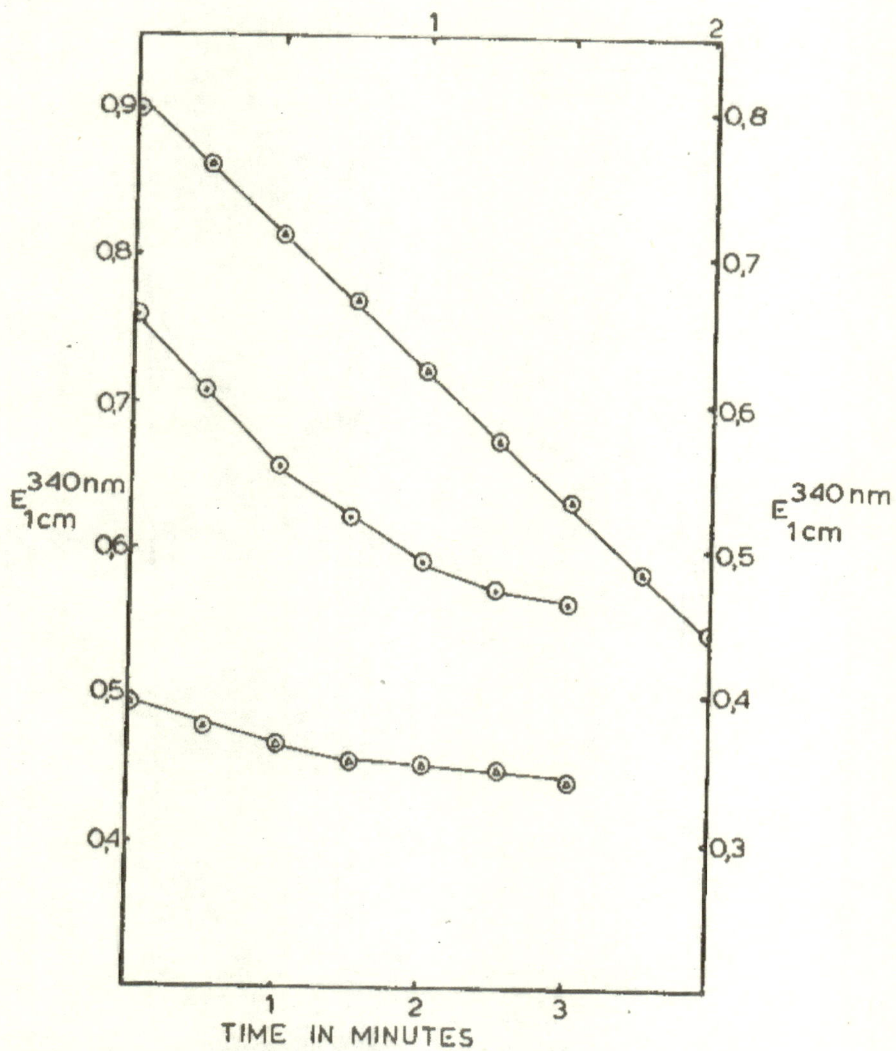

Fig.23: ETP: SPECTROPHOTOMETRIC ASSAY CURVES OF NADH-CoQ_6, NADH-CoQ_{10} AND NADH-MENADIONE REDUCTASE ACTIVITIES

⊙: CoQ_6 reductase
⊙: CoQ_{10} reductase
⊙: menadione reductase

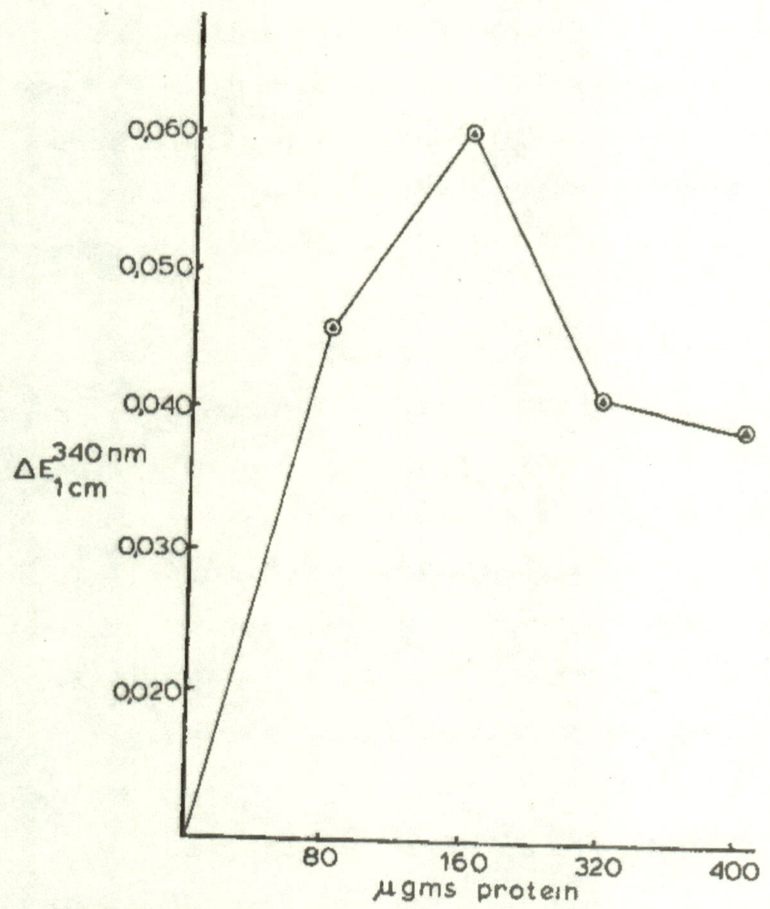

Fig:24: ETP: EFFECT OF PROTEIN CONCENTRATION IN UBIQUINONE COUPLED NADH DEHYDROGENASE

do with the availability of active enzyme sites to the relatively insoluble lipid electron acceptors (COQ_6 and CoQ_{10}). Sanadi found no similar dependence on protein concentration when the water-soluble analogue Menadione was employed as electron acceptor.

Inhibitory studies on NADH-CoQ_6 reductase and on NADH-CoQ_{10} reductase were conducted with 160 µgms of enzyme. In other spectrophotometric assays, a quantity of enzyme was chosen which was capable of producing a rate of change of optical density of 0,10 - 0,15 optical density units per minute.

NADH-Cyt.c. reductase, NADH-CoQ_{10} reductase and NADH-CoQ_6 reductase are all powerfully inhibited by concentrations of halothane below 5mM, whereas NADH-Menadione reductase and NADH-ferricyanide reductase were depressed by less than 10% at this level. The former three assays exhibited the usual type of inhibitory curve (Fig. 25), but with Menadione or ferricyanide as electron acceptor, there is an impression of a sigmoid curve, betokening, in these latter two assays at least, a complex mechanism of inhibition.

Table 16. .../

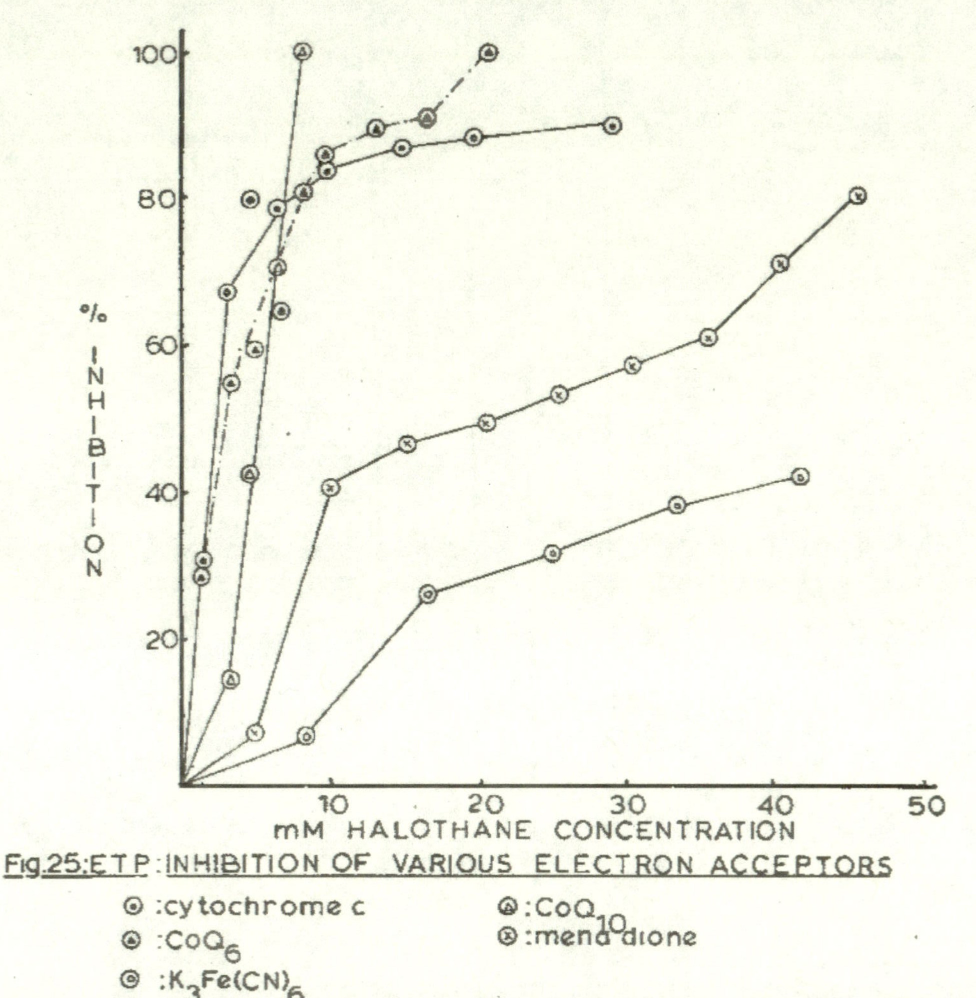

Fig.25: ETP: INHIBITION OF VARIOUS ELECTRON ACCEPTORS

Table 16. The Action of Halothane on ETP NADH Dehydrogenase Linked with Various Electron Acceptors.

Cyt.c.			Menadione			$K_3Fe(CN)_6$		
Halothane	v	% Inhibition	Halothane	v	% Inhibition	Halothane	v	% Inhibition.
-	0,218	0	-	0,131	0	-	0,162	0
1,6	0,150	31	5,0	0,122	7	8,3	0,151	7
3,2	0,070	68	10,0	0,079	40	16,6	0,120	26
4,8	0,044	80	15,0	0,069	47	24,9	0,110	32
6,4	0,048	78	20,0	0,066	50	33,2	0,100	38
9,6	0,035	84	25,0	0,060	54	41,5	0,092	43
14,4	0,028	87	30,0	0,055	58			
19,2	0,026	88	35,0	0,050	62			
28,8	0,020	91	40,0	0,037	72			
76,8	0,004	98						

CoQ_6			CoQ_{10}		
Halothane	v	% Inhibition	Halothane	v	% Inhibtion
-	0,091	0	-	0,087	0
1,6	0,066	28	1,6	0,095	-9
3,2	0,041	55	3,2	0,074	15
4,8	0,036	60	4,8	0,049	44
6,4	0,032	65	6,4	0,026	70
8,0	0,018	81	8,0	0,00	100
9,6	0,012	86			
12,8	0,010	90			
16,0	0,008	91			
20,0	0,0	100			

Each figure is the mean of 3 - 4 experiments.

v : Specific activity.minute $^{-1}$.

Since the assay of the ferricyanide-linked reductase has been shown to be protein-dependent, and since this system was less sensitive to halothane than the naturally-occurring acceptor systems, the inhibitory action of halothane on NADH-ferricyanide reductase was studied at two levels of enzyme protein. (Table 17, Fig. 26). A significantly greater degree of inhibition was observed when 16 µgms of enzyme protein were used in the reaction mixture, instead of 8µgms. Nevertheless, the degree of inhibition still did not approach that exerted by halothane on the Cyt.c., CoQ_6 and CoQ_{10}-linked reductions.

Table 17. Inhibition of NADH-Ferricyanide Reductase by Halothane in Relation to Quantity of Enzyme Protein Present.

mM	v	% Inhibition 8µgms	v	% Inhibition 16µgms
0	0,201	0	0,112	-
8,3	0,187	7	0,076	32
16,6	0,149	26	0,071	37
24,9	0,137	32	0,053	53
33,2	0,125	38		
41,5	0,116	43		

v = enzymic activity. minute^{-1}.

In .../

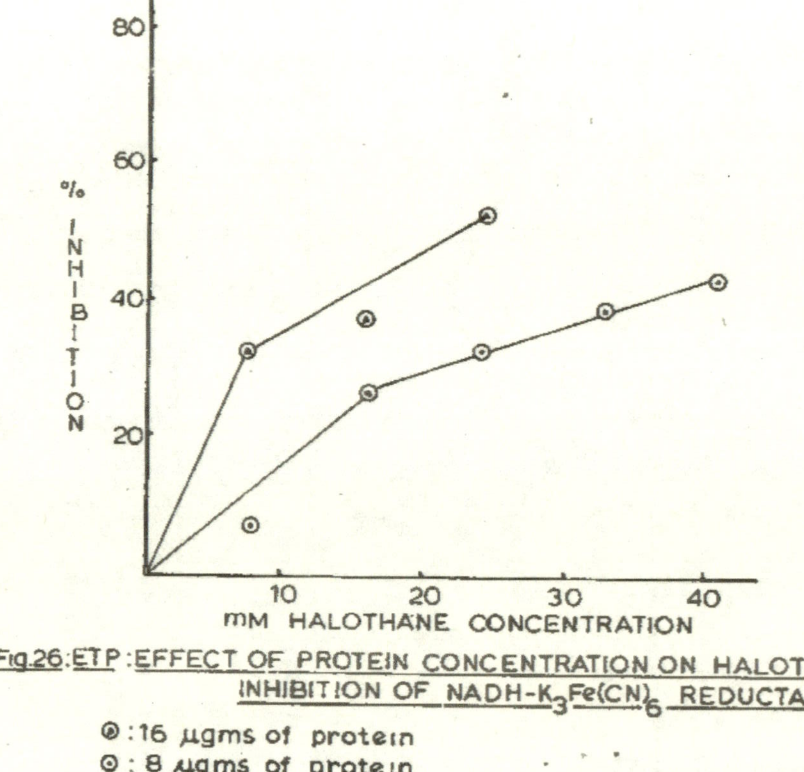

Fig.26: ETP: EFFECT OF PROTEIN CONCENTRATION ON HALOTHANE INHIBITION OF NADH-$K_3Fe(CN)_6$ REDUCTASE

⊙ : 16 µgms of protein

⊙ : 8 µgms of protein

In order to substantiate further the varying susceptibility of NADH dehydrogenase to halothane inhibition, a study was made on natural and artificial electron acceptors at concentrations of halothane of 5 and 10 mM. (Table 18.). The results of this set of experiments clearly demonstrate that reduction of ferricyanide and of menadione by NADH is relatively insensitive to inhibition.

Table 18. Inhibition of a Number of NADH-Linked Redox Systems by 5 and 10 mM Halothane.

Electron Acceptor	% Inhibition.	
	5mM Halothane	10mM Halothane
$K_3Fe(CN)_6$	4	11
Menadione	7	40
CoQ_{10}	48	100
CoQ_6	65	87
Cyt.c.	75	84

Ethanol-Extracted NADH-Dehydrogenase.

Ethanol-extracted NADH-dehydrogenase was assayed by means of the NADH-Cyt.c. reductase method. This enzyme, in the particulate form, had been shown to be sensitive to halothane. The results in Table 19 indicate no inhibition at 10mM halothane, whilst 50% inhibition of the enzyme only occurred at 80mM concentration of the inhibitor.

Table 19. .../

Table 19. Inhibition of Ethanol-Extracted NADH-Cyt.c. Reductase by Halothane.

Halothane mM	Specific Activity	% Activity
0	0,468	100
10	0,472	101
20	0,376	80
40	0,295	63
80	0,239	51

Specific Activity = enzymic activity. mg protein^{-1}.

A comparison of the effects of halothane on the ethanol-extracted and particulate-bound enzyme is shown in Fig. 27, and it can be seen that the solubilised enzyme is much less sensitive to halothane than the intact or native enzyme. In a similar experiment, solubilised NADH-Cyt.c. reductase was prepared from ETP and exposed to halothane. The particulate enzyme was inhibited 95% by 20mM halothane, whereas the extracted soluble form was only 20% inhibited by this concentration of halogenated hydrocarbon. (Table 20). Menadione and ferricyanide reductases were equally inhibited (31%). (Table 20).

Table 20. .../

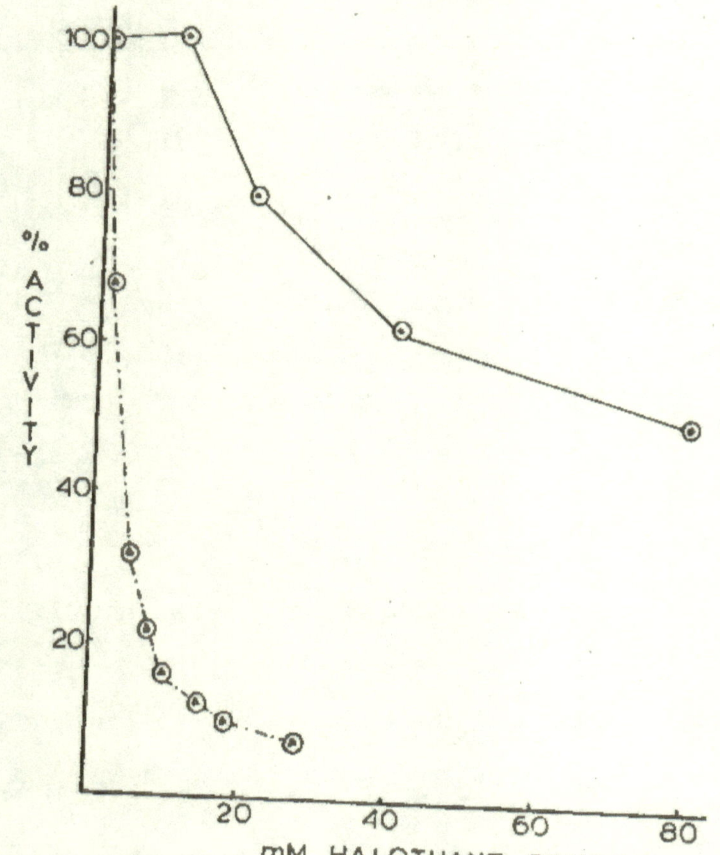

Fig.27: EFFECT OF HALOTHANE ON PARTICULATE AND SOLUBILISED NADH-CYT.C. REDUCTASE

⊙:solubilised preparation of NADH-cyt.c. reductase

⊙:particulate NADH-cyt.c. reductase

Table 20. Inhibition of Particulate and Solubilised Enzyme Preparations by Halothane and Amytal.

Source	Treatment	% Inhibition	Inhibitor mM
ETP	NADH-Cyt.c. reductase	95	20 H.
ETP	NADH-Cyt.c. reductase	71	3 A.
Extract	NADH-Cyt.c. reductase	20	20 H.
Extract	NADH-Cyt.c. reductase	40	3 A.
Extract	NADH-Menadione reductase	31	20 H.
Extract	Ferricyanide reductase	31	20 H.

H : Halothane.

A : Amytal.

Amytal (3mM) likewise caused greater inhibition (71%) of NADH-Cyt.c. reductase within intact ETP than of the ethanolic extract of the enzyme (40%). This finding is in agreement with the observations of Pharo *et al* (1968).

SUMMARY.

The purpose of this investigation was to determine the site of action of halothane and other halogenated hydrocarbons in HBHM and submitochondrial particles, and perhaps to try and shed some light on their mode of action.

From polarigraphic studies, it was established that oxidation of NADH-linked substrates and NADH were sensitive to low concentrations of halothane and other halogenated compounds. NADH oxidase activity of ETP was more than 90% inhibited at less than 2mM halothane. Inhibition of NADH oxidase was reversible at low concentrations of halothane, but irreversible at concentrations greater than 2mM. Inhibitions at both levels, however, could be overcome by the addition of 10mM succinate. This fact proves that the site of inhibition is prior to the point of entry of succinate into the electron transfer chain. In addition, kinetic studies on NADH oxidase activity at varying concentrations of inhibitor led to elucidation of the type of inhibition as uncompetitive. K_{NADH} was determined as 1,60mM, and Ki for halothane was 0,14mM. A series of halogenated compounds inhibited NADH oxidase in a manner similar to that of halothane, whereas the enzyme system was

relatively .../

relatively insensitive to diethyl ether.

Spectrophotometric measurements of NADH oxidation by various electron acceptors revealed specific inhibition of NADH-Cyt.c., NADH-CoQ_6 and NADH-CoQ_{10}-linked reductases by 3mM halothane to the extent of more than 80%. The fact that ferricyanide, assumed to be in equilibrium with the NHI of NADH dehydrogenase, was relatively insensitive to halothane, indicates that the inhibitory site is on the oxygen side of NHI of the flavoprotein complex.

Similar resistance of the water-soluble Menadione, a homologue of CoQ_{10}, underlines the importance of the lipid solubility of the higher ubiquinone analogues, which is related to the length of their side chain.

Solubilised or membrane-free preparations of NADH dehydrogenase, when assayed as NADH-Cyt.c. reductase, were relatively insensitive to the presence of halothane. 3mM halothane inhibited membrane-bound NADH dehydrogenase in ETP by 50%, whereas 80mM was required to produce a similar deleterious effect on the solubilised preparations. This is regarded as evidence that the mitochondrial membrane plays an important role in the action of halogenated and possibly other inhibitors of mitochondrial electron transport.

DISCUSSION .../

DISCUSSION.

Initial studies on the oxidation of NADH or NADH-linked substrates proved that their oxidation was sensitive to low concentrations of halothane as an inhibitor. This inhibition could be overcome by the addition of succinate, indicating that the site of inhibition was prior to the point of entry of succinate into the electron transfer chain, but after the coupling of NAD^+ to its electron donors, whether they be NADH or NADH-linked substrates, since all studies reported showed a selective action of halothane on NADH-mediated oxygen uptake.

These findings are in agreement with the effects of halothane on rat liver mitochondria and HBHM as reported by Harris et al (1971). Miller and Hunter (1970), in their studies on electron transport and oxidative phosphorylation in rat liver mitochondria showed that, at low concentrations of halothane, there was a rapidly reversible effect on electron transport in the region of NADH dehydrogenase. Oxidation of succinate was not affected. At high concentration there was an uncoupling effect, in addition to a partial inhibition of succinate oxidation. At these high concentrations the effect of halothane was irreversible; Harris et al (1971) have studied the action of halothane on HBHM, and found that at low concentrations (< 2mM) oxidation of NADH-linked substrates, but not of succinate,

are .../

are markedly suppressed by halothane. This inhibition was completely reversible.

If one accepts that Coenzyme Q is in the pathway of electron transport, and not on a side chain, the inhibitory action of halothane can be sited somewhere between NADH and CoQ, i.e. in the NADH dehydrogenase complex. The fact that NADH-Cyt.c. reductase activity is also particularly sensitive to halothane, supports this view. There is, however, anomalous behaviour between NADH dehydrogenase activity, when coupled to the naturally occurring CoQ_6 and CoQ_{10} analogues and Menadione. The former activities are inhibited, whereas the Menadione Reductase is not. A similar anomaly has been noted in the study of other inhibitors of NADH dehydrogenase such as Rotenone, Amytal and Piericidin A. The anomaly has been explained by the fact that Menadione is a water-soluble electron acceptor, unlike the lipid soluble, natural acceptors, and is therefore, free to accept electrons along unphysiological pathways. The differences in lipid solubility are thought to be due to differences in the length of the side-chains. There is also the theoretical possibility that Menadione is not in equilibrium with the CoQ component of the electron transfer chain.

The site of inhibition could thus be either on the substrate side or the oxygen side of the flavoprotein-NHI portion of the NADH dehydrogenase complex. Since NADH-

ferricyanide .../

ferricyanide reductase is not inhibited by halothane, and since the artificial electron acceptor, ferricyanide, is thought to be in equilibrium with the NHI portion of the flavoprotein complex, it suggests that the site of inhibition is distal to NHI, i.e. on the oxygen side of the flavoprotein. Similar arguments have been used to place the site of inhibition of the other inhibitors of this complex on the oxygen side of the flavoprotein. It would appear, then, that all known inhibitors of the NADH dehydrogenase have a similar ~~point~~ site of action.

Halothane differs from the other NADH dehydrogenase inhibitors, in that it is volatile and the inhibition can be shown to be relieved reversibly, at least at low concentrations. This is in contrast to the effects of Rotenone and Piericidin A, which bind readily to the NADH dehydrogenase at a number of binding sites with different affinities. Rotenone and Piericidin A can be removed from some of these sites by washing with Bovine Serum Albumin (BSA). The BSA-insensitive sites are thought to be the specific sites responsible for the inhibitory action. It seems that the mode of action of halothane is different in some way from that of the non-volatile inhibitors.

We understand competitive inhibition to mean competition between substrate and inhibitor for the same binding site on the enzyme. In non-competitive inhibition the inhibitor affects the enzyme in such a way that the affinity for the substrate is decreased, and thus the velocity of reaction and the release of substrate to form products, is diminished. In uncompetitive inhibition, however, the binding of substrate to enzyme is not affected, and the inhibition is thought by us to be due to a decrease in the availability of reactive enzyme sites for substrate combination.

It has been shown by kinetics in this study, that the mode of enzyme inhibition is of the uncompetitive type, in that both K_{NADH} and $V_{max.}$ were affected at varying inhibitor concentrations. The plot of 1/v vs 1/c at these varying inhibitor concentrations gave graphs similar to those in Mahler and Cordes (1967). The kinetic parameter for uncompetitive inhibition is that Lineweaver Burk plots at varying inhibitor concentrations give parallel slopes with varying intercepts.

There are several possible explanations of uncompetitive inhibition by halothane. The first is that there is progressive inhibition of the enzyme at one site, in which there is only one pathway of oxidation of NADH dehydrogenation. The second possibility is that there is a single substrate, which is being oxidised by alternate pathways, but still by the same enzyme. Thus, the first site of action of the

enzyme .../

enzyme may be more specifically inhibited than the next, and so on. This involves a progressive inhibition of the enzyme pathways in which the inhibitor sites are saturated in turn, until total inhibition occurs. This mode of inhibition may be accounted for by uncompetitive inhibition, and would point to, and support, the idea of multiple pathways for NADH oxidation.

The third possibility is that halothane induces a type of conformational change in the membrane of the mitochondrion itself, thus altering the availability of the reactive sites to the substrate. The work of Green et al (1970) has shown that conformational changes are possible, and readily occur during the various energy transition states of the mitochondrion. It may be relevant to this concept that, in the reduced state, the mitochondrial NADH dehydrogenase was less sensitive to halothane inhibition than in the oxidised form.

At present it is not possible to decide between the alternatives listed above. The results obtained in this study indicate that the oxidation of added NADH is more sensitive to halothane than that generated by the respective NADH-linked dehydrogenases on their respective substrates. It has been said that mitochondria, generally, are impermeable to NADH. It is, however, a widespread observation that HBHM, when freshly prepared, readily oxidise exogenous NADH.

This .../

This finding has been suggested to be due to damage of the mitochondrial membrane during the isolation procedure. Smoly (1970) concludes that, since mitochondria readily catalyse the oxidation of exogenous NADH via the respiratory chain, it follows that these NADH nucleotides must be localised so that they can easily reach the inside surface of the inner membrane (matrix space). This is supported by the observations of Ernster (1969), who found that the mitochondrial outer compartment is freely permeable to external NADH, and Greenspan (1965), who found that the intramitochondrial NADH nucleotides exchange at a very slow rate with externally-added nucleotides.

Thus the NADH oxidase activity and the greater susceptibility of halothane inhibition of ETP can be explained as being due to the turning inside out of the membrane during sonication. NADH binding sites on the inner side of the inner membrane would, thus, be exposed directly to the action of an inhibitor. The fact that the solubilised enzyme is not inhibited, is further evidence in support of a membrane (conformational) participation in the mode of inhibition of halothane.

The reason for the selectivity of the halogenated compounds at the NADH dehydrogenase step, remains to be elucidated. It is possible that the lipid solubility

of .../

of these compounds is important in this respect, and that they are concentrated at the lipid membrane interface, where they produce their inhibitory effect. This still does not explain the lack of an effect on the succinate pathway. The other factor that appears to be of importance is the degree of halogenation of the compound. As seen from the results, the highly halogenated hydrocarbons are the most potent inhibitors. Carbon tetrachloride has been studied with respect to its hepato-toxicity and cellular damage, which result from peroxidase-type reactions with membrane systems (Slater 1971), consequent to the formation of the free radical $CCl_3^{\cdot}$. Such a mechanism could account for the inhibitory effect of the halogenated hydrocarbons at high concentrations,but cannot explain its reversibility at low concentrations.

The inhibition of halothane and other fluorinated hydrocarbons may be related to their critical surface tension. This group of compounds is known to have particularly low surface tension, in fact they have some of the lowest critical surface tension values which have been determined (Patrick 1971). This would affect their ability to spread over and be absorbed into membranes, where they might produce inhibition. Halothane has a high affinity for lipids, as measured by the high ratio of

oil .../

oil to water (Dundee, 1959), and possibly this factor, and its low surface tension would have a predeliction for lipid of membranes, and thus affect any membrane-bound enzyme activity.

In the presence of halothane without substrate, oxygen uptake was negligible. This excludes the possibility that lipid peroxidation contributed to the observed oxygen uptake and its inhibition in the presence of substrate.

The other factor that may be considered here is why, _in vivo_, during anaesthetic conditions, halothane does not inhibit mitochondrial respiration, although the levels achieved during anaesthesia (±2 mM) would be expected to produce at least 50% or more inhibition of respiration of NADH-linked substrates. There is the possibility that the mitochondria, when isolated, do not have the properties that they have in the intact cell. Then, too, the outer mitochondrial membrane may be damaged, as is suggested by the ability to oxidise exogenous NADH.

The inner and outer mitochondrial membranes differ in their permeability and physical properties. Chappell (1968) found that the outer mitochondrial membrane had a lower percentage of cardiolipin, as compared with the inner membrane. The high content of cardiolipin of the

inner .../

inner membrane is presumably related to the NADH dehydrogenase activity, since it has been shown that NADH dehydrogenase activity was released from the inner membrane, and could be correlated with the degree of hydrolysis of cardiolipin of the inner membrane (Awasthi 1970). The different results obtained in our study on intact mitochondria and ETP may be explained on this basis, since 5mM halothane was required to produce 50% inhibition of pyruvate + malate, oxidation in whole mitochondria whereas halothane (± 1mM) produced 80% or more inhibition of NADH oxidase activity of ETP.

The results reported here, and further investigations which are contemplated, may shed some light on the controversy as to whether CoQ is located in the chain of electron transport, or on a side arm. Extraction of the mitochondria, with acetone containing 4% water, removes the ubiquinone, and the particles are then found to have lost their potential for oxidising succinate by molecular oxygen through Cyt.c. Activity is restored by the addition of CoQ_{10} to the system; other ubiquinone and vitamin K have no effect. This indicates that CoQ_{10} forms an essential link between succinate and Cyt.c. (Lester 1961).

Albracht .../

Albracht *et al* (1971) have extracted ubiquinone with n-pentane to give a fraction free of CoQ, designated P. A second CoQ-free heart muscle extract in which there is no succinate oxidase activity was prepared and its activity restored by the addition of P, indicating succinate oxidase activity is possible in the absence of ubiquinone, if a substance present in the pentane extract P is restored to the preparation. The factor P is under investigation. Such evidence leads one to query the existence of ubiquinone on the direct oxidative pathway; is it on a side arm or a *cul de sac*? - a view long championed by Green and co-workers.

There is some evidence for the existence of alternate pathways of electron transport from the flavoprotein dehydrogenase complex to Cyt.c. Two arrangements A and B have been proposed in Fig. 28. Ragan *et al* (1970) have given evidence for the existence of two NHI pools, which favours A. Similar evidence for two separate pools of Cyt. b. have been described by Chance (1970).

To explain the present results halothane could be postulated to act at two sites distal to NHI in order to give the complete inhibitions noted. Storey and Chance (1967), however, believe that the alternate pathways which have been described are artifactual and are produced during isolation procedures, in which the electron transfer complexes are so altered as to be able to couple with

unnatural .../

Fig. 28. Possible Site of Halothane Inhibition.

A.

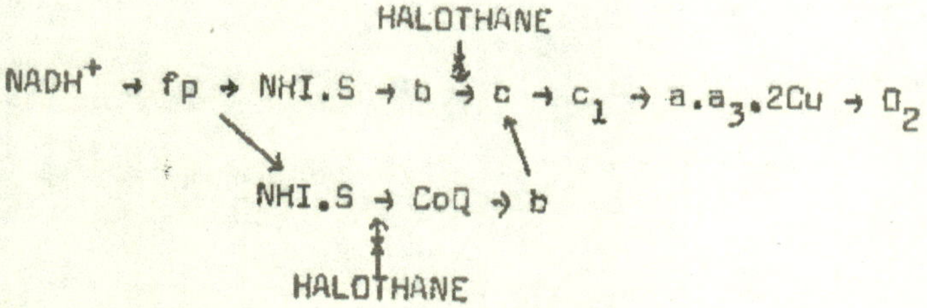

HALOTHANE ↓ (blocked, between b and c)

$NADH^+ \rightarrow fp \rightarrow NHI.S \rightarrow b \rightarrow c \rightarrow c_1 \rightarrow a.a_3.2Cu \rightarrow O_2$

(branch from fp) $\searrow NHI.S \rightarrow CoQ \rightarrow b \nearrow$ (to c)

HALOTHANE ↑ (blocked, at CoQ)

B.

HALOTHANE ↓ (blocked, between fp.NHI.S and c)

$NADH^+ \rightarrow fp.NHI.S \rightarrow c \rightarrow c_1 \rightarrow a.a_3.2Cu \rightarrow O_2$

(branch from fp.NHI.S) $\searrow CoQ \rightarrow b \nearrow$ (to c)

HALOTHANE ↑ (blocked, at CoQ)

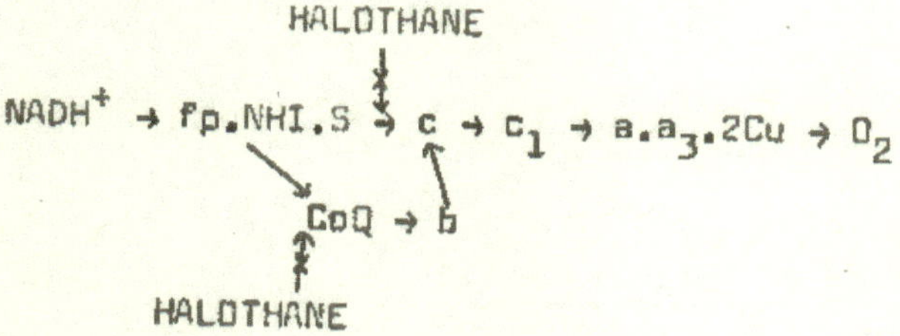

unnatural electron acceptors. Further studies will be necessary to characterise the mode of inhibition of halothane more detail, but it is felt that the model of the particulate-bound NADH dehydrogenase will be suitable for the study of membrane-linked enzymatic reactions in general.

REFERENCES.

-A-

Adriani, J. Editor: Appraisal of Current Concepts in Anesthesiology. 4, 26, 1968.

Albracht, S.P.J., Van Heenkhuizen, H., Slater, E.C., FEBS Letts. 13 No. 5, 265, 1971.

Allaman, D.W., Bachmann, E., Orme-Johnson, N., Tan, W.C., Green, D.E., Arch. Biochem. Biophys. 125, 981, 1968.

Awasthi, Y.C., Ruzicka, F.J., Crane, F.L., Biochem. Biophys. Acta. 203, 233, 1970.

-B-

Berman, M.C., Unpublished Observations. 1969.

Berman, M.C., Harrison, G.G., Bull, A.B., Kench, J.E., Nature London. 225, 653, 1970.

Berman, M.C., Kewley, C.F., Personal Observations. 1970.

Boyer, P.D., Oxidases and Related Redox Systems. Editors: King, T.E., Masson, H.S., Morrison, M. 2, 994, 1965.

Burgos, J., Redfearn, E.R. Biochem. Biophys. Acta. 110, 475, 1965.

Burstein, C., Loyter, A., Racker, E. J. Biol. Chem. 246, 4 075, 1971.

Burstein, C., Kandrach, A., Racker, E. J. Biol. Chem. 246, 4 083, 1971.

-C-

Chapman, A.G., Jagannathan. Scientific Memo 45. Information Exchange Group No. 1. 1963.

Chance, B., Parsons, D.F., Williams, G.R., Ann N.Y. Acad. Sci. 137, 643, 1966.

Chance, B., Erecińska, M., Lee, C.P., Proc. Natl. Acad. Sci. U.S.A., 66, 928, 1970.

Chance, B., Wilson, D.F., Dutton, P.L., Erecińska, M. Proc. Natl. Acad. Sci. U.S.A. 66, 1 175, 1970.

Chappell, J.B., British Med. Bulletin. 24, No. 2, 150, 1968.

Cleland, W.W., Biochem. Biophys. Acta. 67, 104, 1963.

Cleland, W.W., Biochem. Biophys. Acta. 67, 173, 1963.

Cleland, W.W., Biochem. Biophys. Acta. 67, 188, 1963.

Cohen, P.J., Marshall, B.E., Lecky, J. Anaesthesiology. 30, 337, 1969.

Crane, F.L., Glenn, J.L., Green, D.E., Biochem. Biophys. Acta. 22, 475, 1956.

-D-

Dawes, E.A. in Quantitative Problems in Biochemistry. Fourth Edition. Chap. IV. 1967.

De Bernard, B. Biochem. Biophys. Acta. 23, 510, 1957.

Dundee, J.W., in General Anaesthesia. 1, 295, 1959.

-E-

Ernster, L., Luft R., Ikkos, D., Palmieri, G., Afzelius, B. J. Clin. Invest. 41, 1 776, 1962.

Ernster, L., Kuylenstierna, B. in Membranes of Mitochondria and Chloroplasts. 1969.

-F-

Fernandez-Moran, H., Oda, T., Blair, P.V., Green, D.E., J. Cell. Biol. 22, 63, 1964.

-G-

Gornall, A.G., Bardawill, C.H., David, M.M. J. Biol. Chem. 177, 751, 1949.

Green, D.E., Fleischer, S. Horizons in Biochemistry. Albert Szent Gyorgi Dedicatory Vol. Editors: Kasha, M., and Pullman, B. Acad. Press. New York. 1962.

Green, D.E., and Fleischer, S. Biochem. Biophys. Acta. 70, 554. 1963.

Green, D.E., Perdue, J.F., Ann. N.Y.Acad. Sci. 137, 667, 1966.

Green, D.E., Allaman, D.W., Harris, R.A., Tan, W.C., Biochem. Biophys. Res. Commun. 31, 368, 1968.

Green, D.E., Baum H. in Energy and the Mitochondrion. Acad. Press. New York. 1970.

Greenspan, M.D., Purvis, J.L., Biochem. Biophys. Acta. 99, 191, 1965.

Gutman, M., Singer, T.P., Casida, J.E. J.Biol. Chem. 245, 1 992, 1970.

Gutman, M., Singer, T.P., Beinert, H., Casida, J.E. Proc. Natl. Acad. Sci. U.S.A. 65, 763, 1970.

-H-

Hall, C., Wu, M., Crane, F.L., Takahashi, H., Tamura, S., Folkers, K. Biochem. Biophys. Res. Commun. 25, 373, 1966.

Harris, E.J., van Dam, K., Pressman, B.C. Nature London. 213, 1 126, 1967.

Harris, R.A., Penniston, J.T., Asai, J., Green, D.E. Proc. Natl. Acad. Sci. U.S.A. 59, 830, 1968.

Harris, R.A., Munroe, J., Farmer, B., Kim, K.C., Jenkins, P. Arch. Biochem. Biophys. 142, 435, 1971.

Hatefi, Y., Jurtshuk, P., Haavik, A.G. Arch. Biochem. Biophys. 94, 148, 1961.

Hatefi, Y., Haavik, A.G., Jurtshuk, P. Biochem. Biophys. Acta. 52, 106, 1961.

Hatefi, Y., Jurtshuk, P., Haavik, A.G. Biochem. Biophys. Acta. 52, 119, 1961.

Hatefi, Y., Haavik, A.G., Griffiths, D.E. J. Biol. Chem. 237, 1 676, 1962.

Hatefi, Y., Haavik, A.G., Griffiths, D.E. J. Biol. Chem. 237, 1 681, 1962.

Hatefi, Y., Haavik, A.G., Fowler, L.R., Griffiths, D.E., J. Biol. Chem. 237, 2 661, 1962.

Hatefi, Y. Proc. Natl. Acad. Sci. U.S.A. 60, 733, 1968.

Horgan, D.J., Singer, T.P., Casida, J. J. Biol. Chem. 243, 834, 1968.

Horgan, D.J., Palmer, G., Tisdale, H., Singer, T.P., Beinert, H. J. Biol. Chem. 243, 844, 1968

Horgan, D.J., Ohno, H., Singer, T.P., Casida, J.E. J. Biol. Chem. 243, 5 967, 1968.

-J-

Jeng.M., Crane, F.L., Biochem. Biophys. Res. Commun. 32, 945, 1968.

-K-

Kagawa, Y., Racker, E., J.Biol. Chem. 241, 2 475, 1966.

Keilin, D. Proc. Roy. Soc. 104, 206, 1929.

Keilin, D., Hartree, E.F., Biochem. J. 44, 205, 1949.

King, T.E., Howard, R.L., J. Biol. Chem. 236, 1 686, 1962.

King, T.E. in Flavins and Flavoproteins. Editor: Slater, E.C., Amsterdam Elsevier. Page 441. 1966.

King, T.E. Advan. Enzymol. 28, 155, 1966.

King, T.E. Methods in Enzymology X, 202, 1967.

King, T.E., Howard, R.L. Methods in Enzymology X, 275 - 294, 1967.

Klingenberg, M. in Biological Oxidation. Page 3. Editor: Singer, T.P. Interscience 1968.

Klingenberg, M., Palmieri, F., Quagliariello, E., Europ. J. Biochem. 17, 230, 1970

Klingenberg, M. Essays in Biochemistry. 6, 119, 1970.

Kopaczyk, K., Asai, J., Allamann, D.W., Oda, T., Green, D.E. Arch. Biochem. Biophys. 123, 602, 1968.

Korman, E.F., Harris, R.A., Williams, C.M., Green, D.E., Valdiva, E. submitted to J. Bioenerg.

-L-

Lardy, H.A., Ferguson, S.M., Ann. Rev. Biochem. 38, 991, 1969.

Lester, R.L., Fleischer, S., Biochem. Biophys. Acta. 47, 358, 1961.

Lee, C.P., Federation Proc. 22, 527, 1963.

Lee, C.P., Carlsen, K. Federation Proc. 27, 828, 1968.

Lehninger, A.L. in The Mitochondrion. 1965.

Lehninger, A.L. in The Living Cell. Page 85. Readings from Scientific American. 1958 - 1965.

Lipmann, F. Currents in Biochemical Research. Editor: Green, D.E. Page 137. N.Y. Interscience. 1946.

-M-

Machinist, J.M., Singer, T.P., J.Biol. Chem. 240, 3 182, 1965.

Mackler, B., Rao, N.A., Felton, S.P., Huennekens, F.M., J. Biol. Chem. 238, 449, 1963.

Mackler, B., in Flavins and Flavoproteins. Editor: Slater, E.C. Amsterdam Elsevier. 1966.

MacLennan, D.H., Smoly, J., Tzagoloff, A. J. Biol. Chem. 243, 1 589, 1968.

MacLennan, D.H., Tzagoloff, A. Biochem. Biophys. Res. Commun. 33, 441., 1968.

Mahler, H.R., Sarkar, N.K., Vernon, L.P., Alberty, R.A., J. Biol. Chem. 199, 582, 1952.

Mahler, H.R., Cordes, E., in Biological Chemistry. 1967.

Miller, R.N., Hunter, F.E., Mol. Pharmacol. 6, 67, 1970.

Minakami, S., Schindler, F.J., Estabrook, R.W., J.Biol. Chem. 239, 2 042, 1964.

Mitchell, P. Nature. 191, 144, 1961.

Mitchell, P., Moyle, J., Europ. J. Biochem. 9, 149, 1969.

Mockel, J., Dumont, J.E., Europ. J. Clin. Invest. 1, 32, 1970.

-N-

Nicholls, P., Arch. Biochem. Biophys. 106, 25, 1964.

-P-

Palmieri, F., Klingenberg, M. Europ. J. Biochem. 1, 439, 1967.

Patrick, C.R., Chemistry in Britain. 7. No. 4, 154, 1971.

Pharo, R.L., Sanadi, D.R., Biochem. Biophys. Acta. 85, 346, 1964.

Pharo, R.L., Sordahl, L.A., Vyas, S.R., Sanadi, D.R. J. Biol. 241, 4 771, 1966.

Pharo, R.L., Sordahl, L.A., Edelhock, H., Sanadi, D.R. Arch. Biochem. Biophys. 125, 416, 1968.

-R-

Ragan, C.I., Clegg, R.A., Haddock, B.A., Light, P.A., Garland, P.B. FEBS Letts. 8, 333, 1970.

Redfearn, E.R., King, T.E., Nature London. 202, 1 313, 1964.

Rieske, J.S., Hansen, R.E., Zaugg, W.S., J. Biol. Chem. 239, 3 017, 1964.

Rieske, J.S., Zaugg, W.S., Hansen, R.E. J. Biol. Chem. 239, 3 023, 1964.

Ringler, R.L., Minakami, S., Singer, T.P. J. Biol. Chem. 238, 801, 1963.

-S-

Salach, J., Singer, T.P., Bader, P. J. Biol. Chem. 242, 4 555, 1967.

Sanadi, D.R., Ann. Rev. Biochem. 34, 21, 1965.

Sanadi, D.R., Pharo, R.L., Sordahl, L.A. Methods in Enzymology X, 297, 1967.

Schnaitman, C., Greenawalt, J.W., J. Cell. Biol. 38, 158, 1968.

Singer, T.P. in Biological Oxidation. Page 339. Editor: Singer, T.P. Interscience. 1968.

Slater, E.C., Nature. 172, 975, 1953.

Slater, E.C., Mitochondria: Structure and Function. Editor: Ernster, L. London Academic. 17, 205, 1969.

Slater, T.F., Sawyer, B.C. Biochem. J. 123, 805, 1971.

Smith, A. Methods in Enzymology X, 81, 1967.

Smoly, J., Kuylenstierna, B., Ernster, L. Proc. Natl. Acad. Sci. U.S.A. 66, 125, 1970.

Stier, A., Alter, H., Hessler, O., Rehder, K. Anesth. Analg. 43, 723, 1964.

Stier, A. Biochem Pharmacol. 13, No. 1, 544, 1964.

Storey, B.T. Arch. Biochem. Biophys. 121, 261, 1967.

Storey, B.T. Arch. Biochem. Biophys. 121, 271, 1967.

Storey, B.T., Chance, B., Arch. Biochem. Biophys. 121, 279, 1967.

-T-

Teeter, M.E., Baginsky, M.L., Hatefi, Y. Biochem. Biophys. Acta. 172, 331, 1969.

Tyler, D.D., Butow, R.A., Gonze, J., Estabrook, R.W. Biochem. Biophys. Res. Comm. 19, 551, 1965.

-V-

Vallin, I., Löw, H. Europ. J. Biochem. 5, 402, 1968.

Van Dam, K., Meyer, A.J., Ann. Rev. Biochem. 40, 748, 1971.

Vanderkooi, G., Green, D.E., Proc. Natl. Acad. Sci. U.S.A. 66, 615, 1970.

Vanderkooi, G., Sundaralingam, M. Proc. Natl. Acad. Sci. U.S.A. 67, 233, 1970.

APPENDIX

FORMULAE

ATP (adenosine 5′-triphosphate)

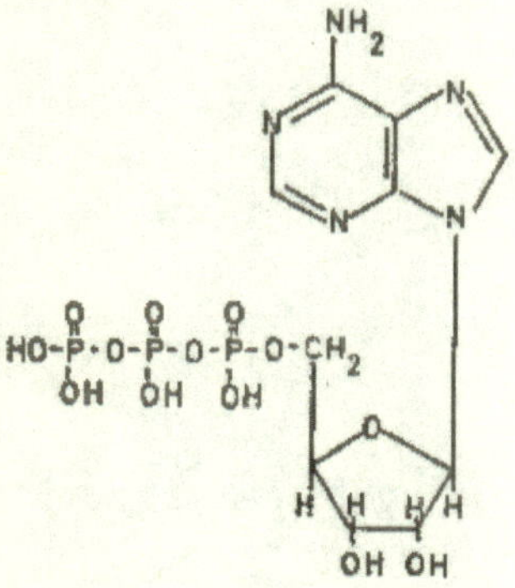

Amytal

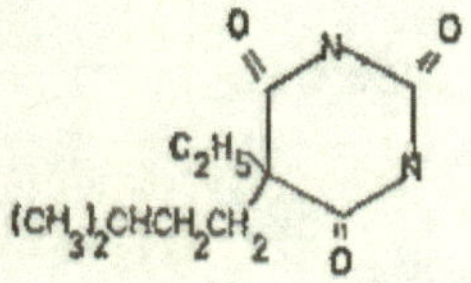

Antimycin $A_1 (C_{28}H_{40}N_2O_9)$

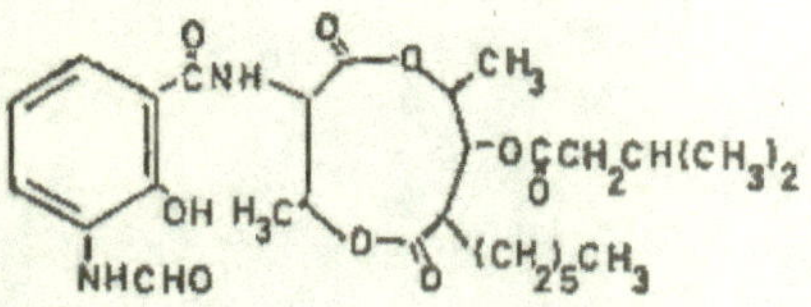

L-Ascorbic acid (L-ascorbate = anion)

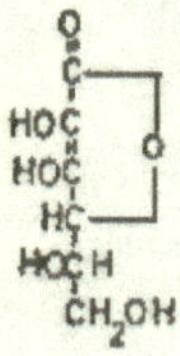

Azide (N_3^-)

$$^-N=\overset{+}{N}=N^-$$

Blastomycin (Antimycin A_3: $C_{26}H_{36}N_2O_9$)

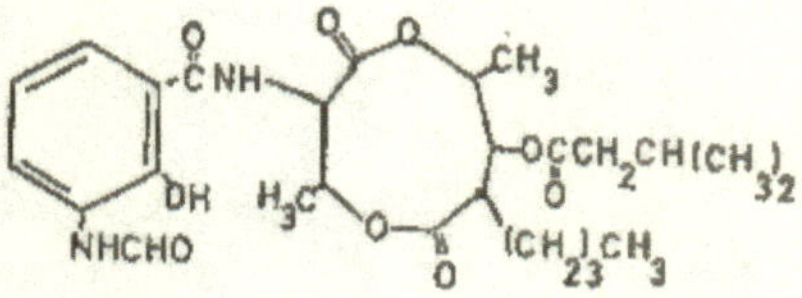

Cardiolipin

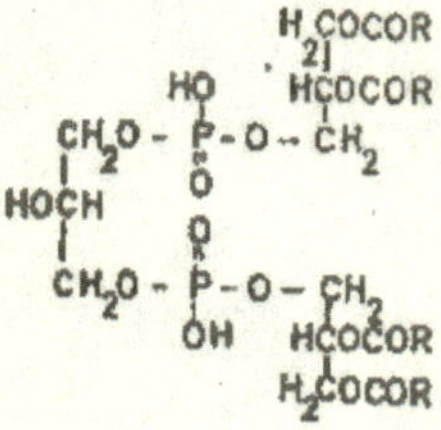

where RCO = acyl group

p-Chloromercuri benzoate (p-CMB)

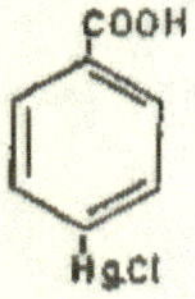

CoQ (Ubiquinone)

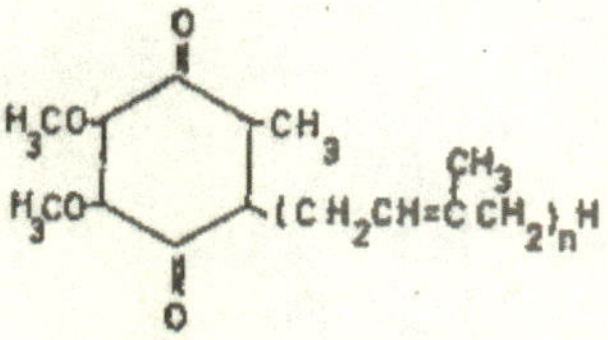

n = 6 for bacteria
n = 10 for beef heart

Cytochromes (Porphyrins of cytochromes A, B, C and D)

A :

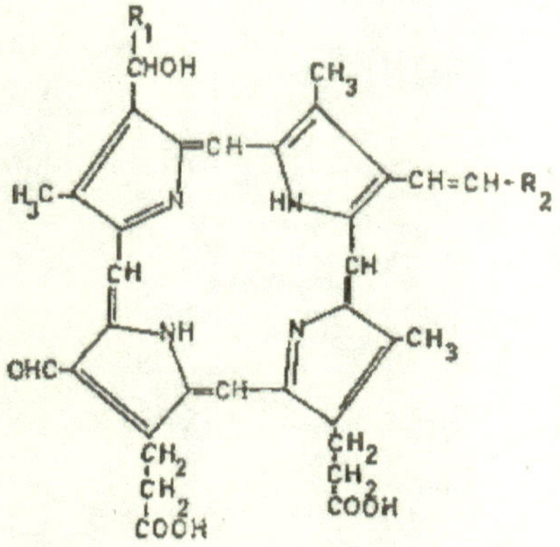

B :

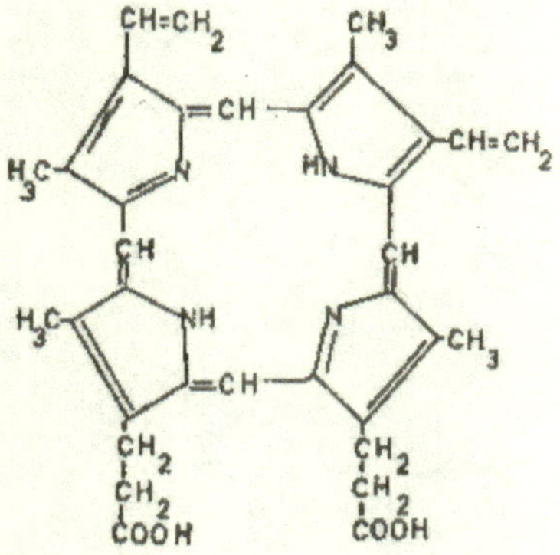

C :

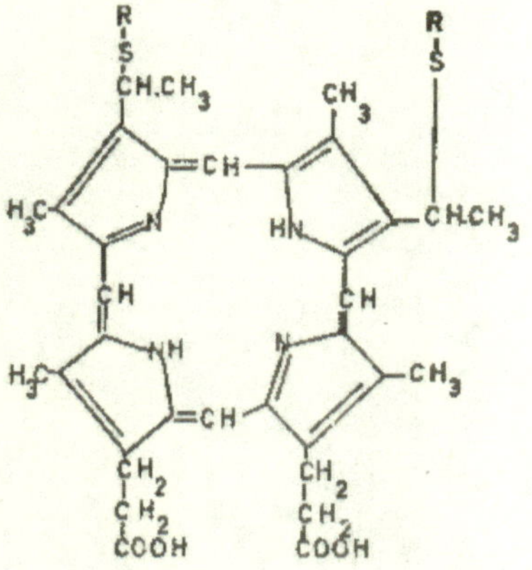

D :

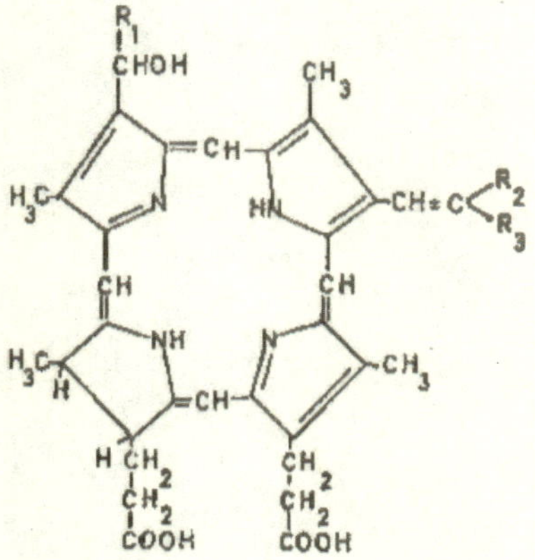

Deoxycholate (DOC : $C_{24}H_{40}O_4$)

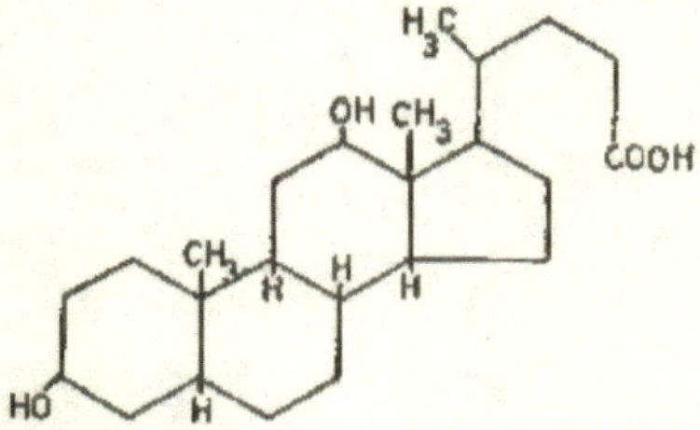

2,6-Dichloroindophenol (DCIP)

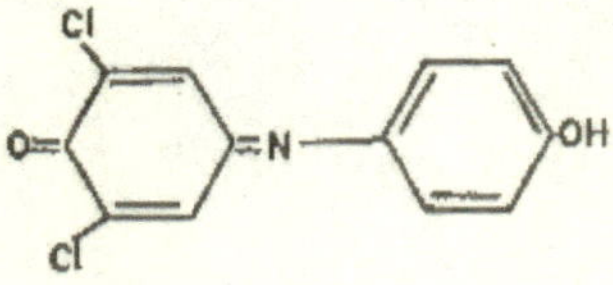

Dicoumarol

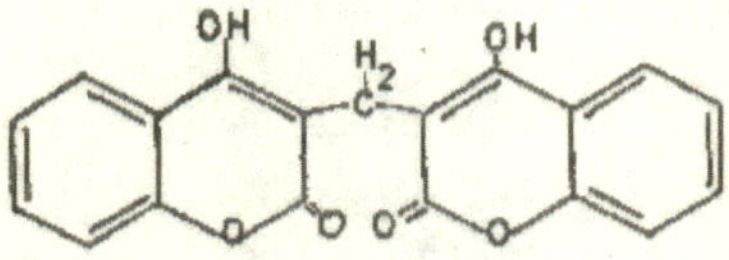

2,4 Dinitrophenol (DNP)

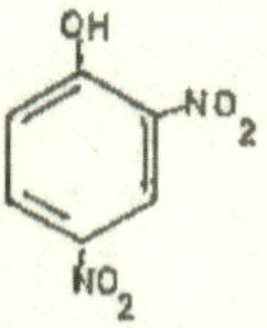

OH
NO_2
NO_2

Ethylenediaminetetraacetic acid (EDTA) disodium salt

$$(CH_2COOH)_2NCH_2CH_2N(CH_2COONa)_2$$

Flavin (oxidized)

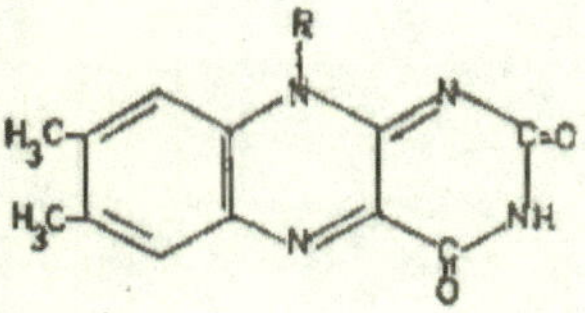

R
N
N
H_3C
C=O
H_3C
NH
N
C
O

FAD (flavin adenine dinucleotide)

R :

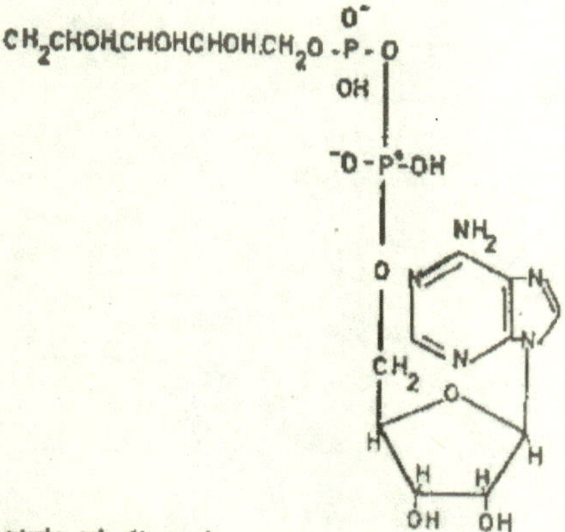

$CH_2CHOHCHOHCHOHCH_2O-P(O^-)(OH)-O$

$^-O-P^*-OH$

O

NH_2

N

N

N

N

CH_2

O

H

H

H

H

OH OH

FMN (flavin mononucleotide, riboflavin)

R :

$CH_2CHOHCHOHCHOHCH_2O-P^*(O^-)(OH)-OH$

Glutamic acid (glutamate : anion)

COOH
|
CH_2
|
CH_2
|
$CHNH_2$
|
COOH

Gramicidin S

L-Leu — D-Phe — L-Pro — L-Val — L-Orn — L-Leu — D-Phe — L-Pro — L-Val — L-Orn — (cyclic)

Halothane (fluothane)

$CF_3CHBrCl$

α-Ketoglutarate (2-oxoglutarate)

COOH
|
CH_2
|
CH_2
|
C=O
|
COOH

Malate = anion (Malic acid)

COOH
|
HOCH
|
CH_2
|
COOH

Malonic acid

COOH
|
CH_2
|
COOH

Menadione (Vit.K_3)

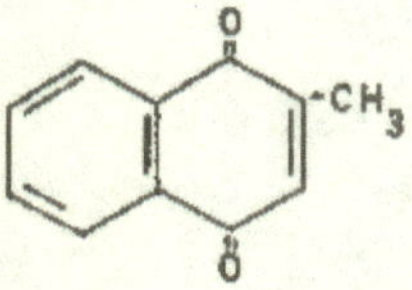

NAD* (nicotinamide adenine dinucleotide)

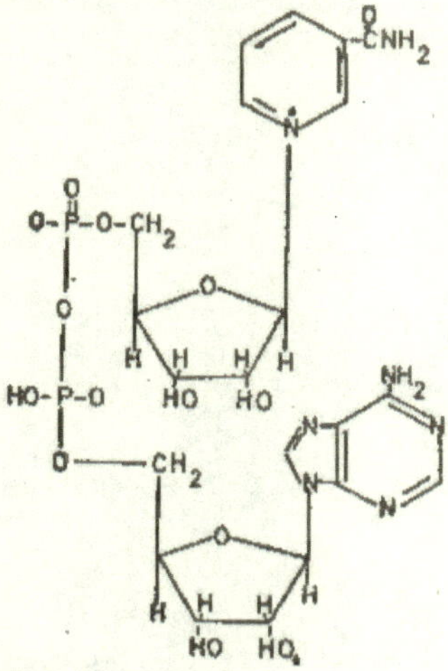

another phosphate group is added here for NADP

NADH

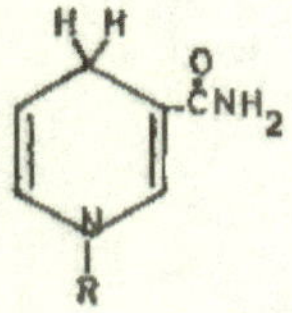

Oligomycin

A : $C_{24}H_{40}O_6$
B : $C_{22}H_{36}O_6$
C : $C_{28}H_{46}O_6$

Piericidin A

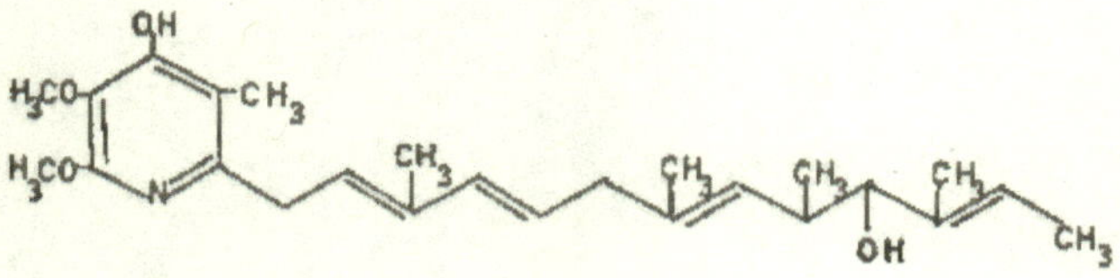

Phosphatidyl choline (α-Lecithin)

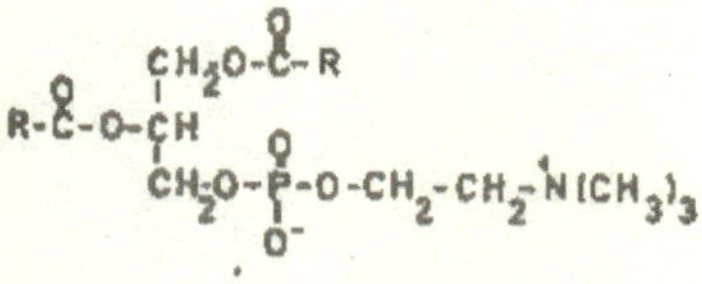

RCO=acyl group

Phosphatidyl ethanolamine (α-Cephalin)

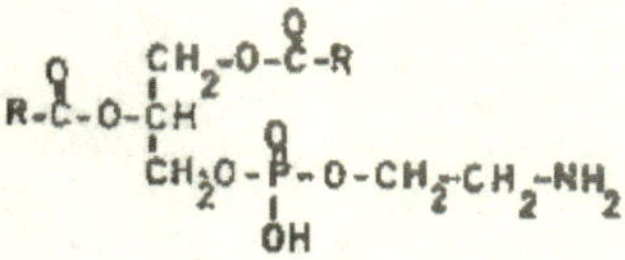

RCO=acyl group

Plastoquinone

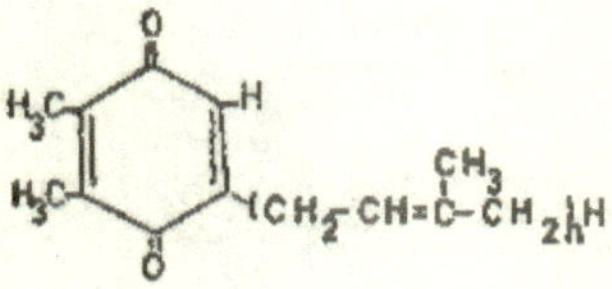

Protoporphyrin IX

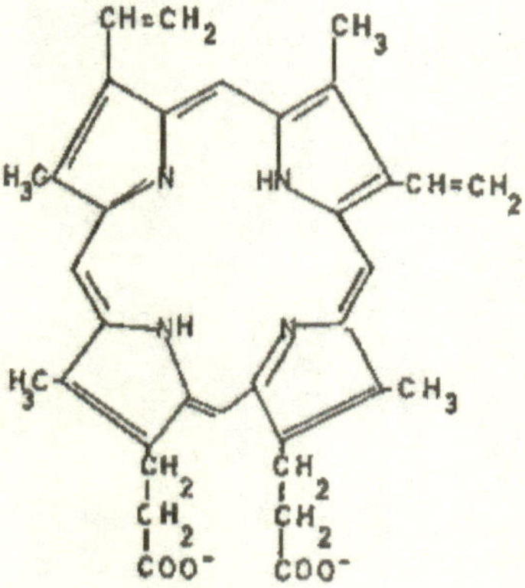

Pyruvic acid (anion = pyruvate)

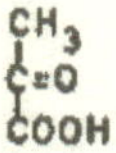

Rotenone

II :

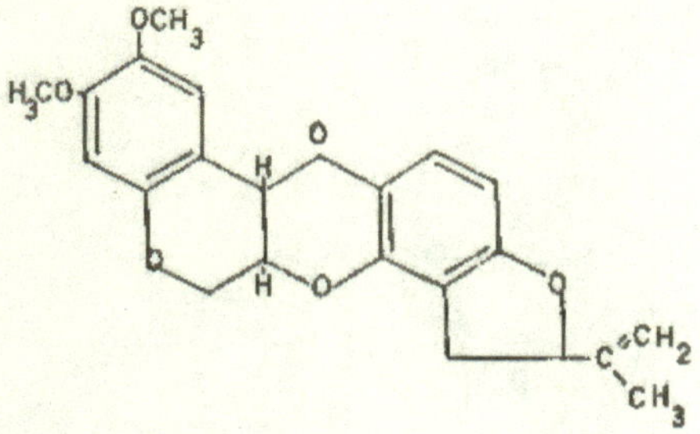

Seconal (secobarbital sodium)

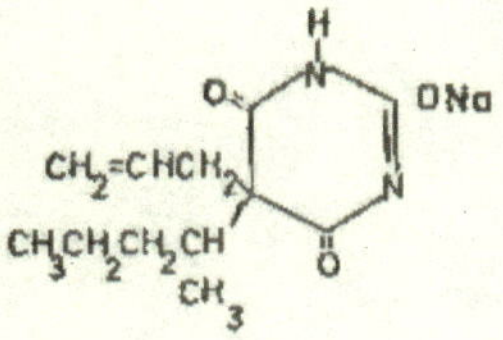

Succinic acid (anion=succinate)

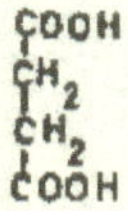

COOH
CH_2
CH_2
COOH

Tartaric acid
(meso)

COOH
CHOH
CHOH
COOH

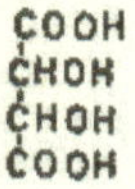

TMPD (tetramethyl-P-phenylenediamine)

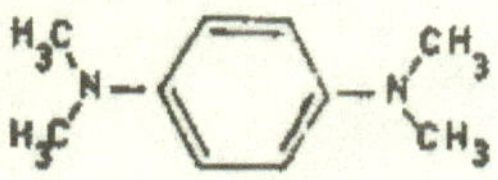

Tris (tromethamine)

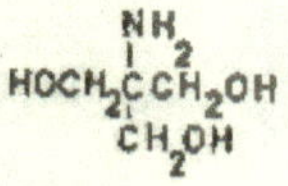

$HOCH_2C(NH_2)(CH_2OH)CH_2OH$

Trifluoroacetic acid

CF_3
COOH

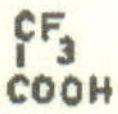

Vitamin K

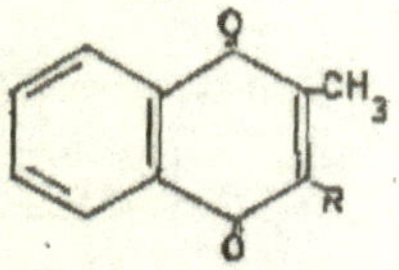

K_1 : R = $-CH_2CH{=}C(CH_3)CH_2(CH_2CH_2CH(CH_3)CH_2)_3H$

K_2 : R = $-(CH_2CH{=}C(CH_3)CH_2)_6H$

www.ingramcontent.com/pod-product-compliance
Lightning Source LLC
La Vergne TN
LVHW090939150826
845672LV00006B/1556